Age Appropriate Activities for Adults with Profound Mental Retardation

A Collaborative Design by Music Therapy,
Occupational Therapy, and Speech Pathology

Nina Galerstein
Kris Martin
Darryl L. Powe

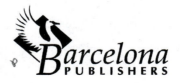

Barcelona
PUBLISHERS

Age Appropriate Activities for Adults with Profound Mental Retardation

ISBN 1-891278-32-0

2 4 6 8 9 7 5 3 1

Distributed throughout the world by:
Barcelona Publishers
4 White Brook Road
Gilsum NH 03448
Tel: 603-357-0236 Fax: 603-357-2073
Website: www.barcelonapublishers.com
SAN 298-6299

Cover design:
© 2005 Frank McShane

Foreword To Second Edition

The second edition of this book (2005) is almost identical to the first. The definitions of our therapeutic practices remain essentially the same, and the activities are still relevant and useful. People with profound mental retardation have the same needs, abilities, similarities, challenges, and unique personalities. Some of the resources in Part III have changed, mostly due to the widespread use of the internet. Interestingly, what has not changed since we began our research in 1995, is the scarcity of practical activities and programs for this population. Therefore, this book is submitted with pleasure for its second printing, and we hope it find its way into the hands of those who really need it.

Nina Galerstein, Kris Martin, Darryl L. Powe

Acknowledgements

The authors would like to express heartfelt appreciation to the people who assisted in the completion of this book: in particular, Susan Nelson, M.Ed., M.S., SLP, who wrote the scenario entitled Turntaking (Throwing a Ball) and Kelly Richardson, C.O.T.A., who wrote the procedures for three scenarios (Homemaking, Plan Care, and Pet Care).

We would also like to acknowledge our colleagues at Stockley Center in Georgetown, Delaware who were members of the original task force from which this project developed: Joseph Keyes, Ph.D., Director of Professional Services, Linda Hare-Tucker, M.A., N.C.C., Behavior Analyst, and Karen Widen, Sheltered Workshop Production Foreman. In addition, our thanks extend to our other colleagues who provided ideas, resources, and support: Pauline Barcus, Mary Kay Henderson, Kimberly Lau, Lori Marshall, Arlene Metz, and Julia Pescor.

We are grateful to Karen D. Hutson for her expertise in word processing and to Jennifer August, M.C.A.T., ATR-BC for the book's illustrations.

Ultimately, we would like to acknowledge with gratefulness all our teachers, mentors, and clients (both past and present) who have taught us, above all, that it is not what we teach our clients, but what our clients teach us.

Contents

INTRODUCTION

BACKGROUND, CLIENTELE, AUDIENCE, APPLICATION

Assessment and treatment programs always present a challenge when clients are developmentally disabled. This challenge increases significantly when the diagnostic level of mental retardation is profound,[1] and the client has multiple disabilities, such as spastic quadriplegia, autism, vision/hearing impairments, and so forth. For these individuals, therapeutic intervention is crucial but often frustrating for both the caregiver and the client.

At our facility, a state residential treatment center for adults with developmental disabilities, a group of therapists were faced with the task of creating a structured habilitation program for sixty individuals with profound mental retardation. These individuals were to be working in groups of four, with twelve to sixteen individuals in each large room. Based on needs, for maximal treatment results, it would have been ideal to provide each person with one-to-one staffing all day. The reality was that this was impossible; each group of four would have one caregiver, and this person would have to provide active treatment[2] to all clients throughout their day. Our group of therapists was asked to design this active treatment program. In addition, our program design had to ensure that all activities were

age appropriate.[3] In other words, these activities needed to be "...designed to teach skills by age-appropriate processes and at age-appropriate times..." and materials needed to be offered to reinforce and reflect age-appropriate behaviors. (Gardner and Chapman, 1990) This presented major challenges due to lack of available materials (instructional, recreational, etc.) for adults who function developmentally at less than one year of age.

Naturally, our first strategy was to attempt to locate any sources that would assist us with our task. We looked through catalogs, visited libraries, consulted with professional colleagues, and networked at conferences. We discovered that most of the existing materials were either for children or for adults with a higher level of functional skills. In addition, if we did find a source that addressed profound mental retardation, it generally referred to those persons who test at the profound level cognitively, but function at a much higher level in social and daily living activities. The clients in our program have multiple challenges that affect every aspect of their daily lives. Most use wheelchairs, have little or no communication skills, have major sensory deficits, and depend upon caregivers to meet all their basic daily living/personal care needs. They are unique people who do have the capacity to learn, yet can be frustrating to work with because of the length of time they

---

(1) 318.2 Profound mental retardation (IQ level below 20 or 25): The group with profound mental retardation constitutes approximately 1% to 2% of people with mental retardation. Most individuals with this diagnosis have an identified neurological condition that accounts for their mental retardation. During the early childhood years, they display considerable impairments in sensorimotor functioning. Optimal development may occur in a highly structured environment with constant aid and supervision and an individualized relationship with a caregiver. Motor development and self care and communication may improve, if appropriate training is provided. Some can perform simple tasks in closely supervised and sheltered settings (DSM IV).

(2) Active treatment is "...the consistent, aggressive, continuous, and accountable application of habilitation interventions by caregivers of persons with developmental disabilities." (Manfredini and Smith, 1988). "Active treatment is based on the premise that all people, regardless of the severity of their disability, grow and develop throughout their lives." (Gardner et al.,1990)

(3) Age appropriateness requires "...that conditions of everyday life be representative of an individual's chronological age (CA) rather than developmental age." (Matson, Sadowski, Matese, Benavidez, 1993)

take to learn. As stated previously, we found that resources for active treatment for adults with profound mental retardation were virtually nonexistent. Therefore, our program design developed as a result of shared expertise in our therapeutic fields—music therapy, occupational therapy, and speech pathology.

We offer this book to those people who are faced with challenges similar to ours. This book is written for teachers, families, therapists, friends, trainers—anyone who works with and/or lives with people with very severe disabilities. We offer activities that are interesting and are fun and which will enhance performance in the completion of functional tasks. These activities are designed to be implemented by any caregiver, and as such, are easy to do and generally require minimal or inexpensive materials. It is important to add that they are all age-appropriate; they are designed specifically for adults and have been successfully implemented with this population.

In addition to these activities, this book offers our definitions of each therapy; when we began our collaboration, we realized that we did not fully understand the scope and details of each other's work. Without this knowledge, we were unable to move forward. We also offer definitions for the specific disabilities that can coexist with mental retardation. These definitions can be helpful and instructive when considering individual needs and activities. In addition, this book addresses common issues for this population, i.e., the concept of group work versus individual programming and the need for developing functional communication. Finally, the book offers both activities and related resources for an interesting and successful program.

We would like to state again that it is our belief that all people with developmental disabilities have the capability of learning and of interacting with other people. It is our task to find the way to foster this learning process for each person. It is certainly a major challenge to work with people that do not provide you with much feedback and for whom every task

must be pared down to the most basic elements. We believe that a collaborative effort, utilizing specially designed activities, can provide a positive experience for both the client and the caregiver.

DEFINITIONS OF THE THERAPIES

Music Therapy

Edith H. Boxill, a Music Therapist who specializes in the treatment of people with developmental disabilities, defines music therapy as "...an amalgam of music and therapy. When music, as an agent of change, is used to establish a therapeutic relationship, to nurture a person's growth and development, to assist in self-actualization, the process is music therapy. Broadly defined, music therapy is the use of music as a therapeutic tool for the restoration, maintenance, and improvement of psychological, mental, and physiological health and for the habilitation, rehabilitation, and maintenance of behavioral, developmental, physical and social skills—all within the context of a client-therapist relationship."

Music Therapy has a lengthy history. The first published article in the United States appeared in1789. This was the same year George Washington was elected President. Throughout the 1800's there were other published accounts of using music to treat various health issues. (Clair, 1996 p. 3-4)

During World War II at veteran's hospitals, the use of music in psychiatric care was applied to address specific need and issues. In 1944, the first university music therapy curriculum was established to train music therapists formally. In 1950, the National Association for Music Therapy was organized, (now the American Music Therapy Association) making possible standardizations of education, clinical training, and clinical practice.

As as member of the team, the professional music therapist assesses needs, plans a course of treatment, and evaluates progress. Music and music activities are specifically selected for use with a particular client, based on the music therapist's knowledge of the effects of music on behavior, and the client's strengths, needs, and goals. Because music is multisensory, it is ideal for use with people with developmental disabilities—it provides auditory, visual, tactile and kinesthetic stimulation. Music activities can provide motivation and opportunities for developing and/or increasing motor, communication, social, cognitive, and leisure/recreation skills. As such, therapeutic music activities can support speech, physical, and occupational therapy programs by providing an alternative treatment modality. Music may also be used in behavioral therapy to increase or modify adaptive behaviors and to extinguish maladaptive/inappropriate behaviors. In these programs, music can be used as positive or negative reinforcement, or a cue for other behaviors.

Occupational Therapy

The name occupational therapy is misleading in today's society when the term occupation refers to job- or career-related issues. Yet the scope of occupational therapy has been much broader ever since its inception in the United States in the early 1900s. Occupational therapy essentially concerns itself with occupational behavior that can be defined as "...an activity in which person engage during most of their waking time; it includes activities that are playful, restful, serious, and productive. These work, play and daily living activities are carried out by individuals in their own unique ways based on their beliefs and preferences, the kinds of experiences they have had, their environments and the specific patterns of behaviors that they acquire over time." (Kielhofner, 1985)

The first practitioners of occupational therapy worked exclusively in the long term psychiatric facilities in this country. Occupational therapy's instrumental belief was to use activity to serve as a motivating and therapeutic influence for persons with either a cognitive or social handicap.

As the profession grew, the events of World War I and World War II had a profound effect on occupational therapy and it's traditional treatment domain of addressing only mental disabilities. With the incorporation of occupational therapy in the military medial corps, the focus was to utilize activity to serve as a diversion for the injured soldiers. Quickly, however, the therapeutic effects of occupational therapy and its prescriptive activities were realized to impact the physical recuperation of the wounded as effectively as it addressed the coginitive or social difficulties of the psychiatric patients. Thus, the evolution of occupational therapy began with settings that treat physical disabilities and this continues to make up the majority of today's occupational therapy clinics.

Change and growth guided the early times of occupational therapy. Modern practitioners would find this statement to ring true even today. It is true that a concise definition of the profession is difficult. The best description of occupational therapy should therefore incorporate the use of multiple statements:

- Occupational therapy is holistic in that it treats persons with an injury or illness that results in either chronic or acute physical, cognitive or social handicaps.

- Occupational therapy works to negate or lessen the effects of these disabilities with patients across the life span—from premature infants to geriatric clients.

- Occupational therapy utilizes activities, especially those stated by the patient to be important or motivating intrinsically, in addition to medicine and/or exercise as part of their treatment.

Speech/Language Pathology

Speech Pathology is the science of diagnosing and treating disorders of communication. At this point, it is important to note that communication, in its purest sense, can be summed up as the exchange of ideas. This exchange can be through speech, through writing, through physical manipulation, and through any other mode by which point A is transmitted to point B. Thus speech/language pathology may be considered the study of treating anything that may inhibit communication between these points.

The previously-mentioned definition may prove rather limiting with respect to the scope of the field itself. The following lists the general type of disorders treated by Speech/language pathologists (SLP's):

Scope of Practice for Speech Pathology

- **Voice:** Aiding singers, professional speakers (newscasters, clergymen, and others) to utilize safer and more efficient vocal practices
- **Fluency:** Also known as stuttering
- **Aphasia:** Language loss or impairment following brain injury
- **Dysarthria/Apraxia:** Speech production difficulties following brain injury
- **Articulation:** Production of sound for the purposes of speech, foreign accent reduction and business dialect enhancement
- **Augumentative/Alternative Communication:** The use of computers and other devices to aid in communication when individuals are unable to speak
- **Aural Rehabilitation:** Helping hearing-impaired individuals utilize social cues to receive messages in compensation for hearing loss.

Speech/language pathologists also work with the following:
- **Language Impairment:** second language acquisition, language and developmental delay, etc.
- **Dyslexia:** Reading disorders

Most recently, SLPs have been working with disorders of deglutition, or swallowing. Such disorders (dysphagia) may result from strokes, brain injury, tongue surgery, etc.

There are three specific periods/eras which encompass the formation of speech pathology as an allied health field. (1) Europe in the period before World War I (WWI) and (2) America between the industrial revolution, and immediately following WWI. The roots of speech pathology began in the mid 1800s during the formative years of psychology in the attempt to understand stuttering. During that period, European psychologists began to explore whether or not stuttering was a psychological disorder. Before then, stuttering had been viewed as a sign of mental illness or an aberrant behavior demonstrated by individuals with mental illness. Also during this period, physicians, during autopsies, began to notice the presence of lesions or injury in the brains of individuals who had previously suffered language impairment following strokes and head injuries.

As an autonomous field speech/language pathology began between the years of the American industrial revolution and World War I and formed itself under the works of Alexander Graham Bell and Pierre Gallaudet. Bell is known for various inventions, e.g., the telephone, phonograph, etc., but he is also credited with the first formation of sign language that he utilized in helping a close relative to communicate. Gallaudet is credited with having established the first generalized teaching program for individuals with hearing impairments.

INTERDISCIPLINARY COLLABORATION

In recent years, the philosophy of medical and educational establishments has changed from a multidisciplinary to an interdisciplinary approach. The multidisciplinary model exists when each discipline, providing treatment for one individual, implements separate and different courses of action. Although these professionals may never consult with or interact with each other, they will interact with the client and/or caregiver. The interdisciplinary approach is more cooperative and interactive.

It mandates that each discipline, providing treatment for one individual, gives feedback to each other for the purposes of collaboration. This collaboration facilitates communication between team members thereby reducing duplication of services and increasing time efficiency and cost-effectiveness. The interdisciplinary approach, with regard to mental retardation, focuses attention on the person as a whole and recognizes that the needs of these people extend beyond the orientation of one discipline. (Gardner, et al., 1990)

In our work, the collaboration of music therapy, occupational therapy, and speech pathology began as a necessity—we were chosen to work together to design the habilitation program described earlier. In the beginning we were not convinced that we could find common ground but soon discovered that our similarities strengthened our differences. Together we could produce functional activities that addressed many different skill areas, and also helped increase the clients' quality of life. Because we believe strongly in the interdisciplinary approach to programming, therapeutic collaboration became natural and exciting. Our philosophy regarding our clients was exactly the same:

- Adults with profound mental retardation are capable of learning, if provided optimal circumstances.

- Adults with profound mental retardation deserve the same opportunities as everyone else.

- Adults with profound mental retardation deserve treatment that is tailored to adult needs, not those of children.

- Adults with profound mental retardation need to be grouped together, based on needs, capabilities, and social/peer preferences.

- Collaborative therapy is a holistic approach and offers clients a variety of interesting choices that can lead to the development of functional skills.

- All professionals working with people with mental retardation essentially speak the same language and effectively fit into one another's modes of treatment.

PART ONE

Populations, Programs, and Communication

Chapter 1

Population Descriptors

This chapter is a listing of descriptors that pertain to persons with profound mental retardation—the target population in this book. These descriptors are intended to provide basic knowledge and vocabulary for a greater understanding of these people and their needs. The definitions are divided into the following skill areas: physical/motor, sensory, and communication. The citations in this chapter are designed to

- *Assist*—caregivers in determining if this resource addresses clients' needs
- *Educate*—the reader to the facets of the profound developmentally disabled population of which they may not be commonly aware
- *Clarify*—the disabilities that make programming difficult for this population

PHYSICAL/MOTOR
Terms that apply to the body and how it moves

Orthopedic: concerning the bones and/or joints of the body
- **Joint Contracture:** when the normal movement of a joint is constricted.
- **Scoliosis:** a curving of the spine to one side or another.
- **Osteoporosis:** a softening or thinning of a bone related to age or disuse.

Neurologic: dealing with the brain and how it controls the body
- **Epilepsy:** a disorder of the nervous system, characterized by convulsions (seizure disorder).
- **Spasticity:** a tightness or rigidity of the muscles so that movement is difficult.
- **Flaccidity:** a laxity or looseness of a muscle.

Movement Disorder: difficulty initiating or controlling motion
- **Athetoid:** involuntary random, flailing movements of head or limbs.
- **Hemiparesis:** paralysis or restricted motion on one side of the body (leg & arm).
- **Paraplegia:** paralysis or restricted motion of lower trunk and/or legs.

SENSORY

Alluding to the five traditional senses (vision, hearing, touch, taste, smell) and the additional senses that provide information about the internal feelings of the body (proprioception, kinesthesia, vestibular)

Visual Impairment: May apply to limitations of the structure of the eye in seeing an image, as well as the ability of the brain to register or attend to the image effectively.

Hearing Impairment: May pertain to a physical problem in the structures of the ear which conduct sound, as well as the inability of the brain to register or attend to the sound accurately.

Sensory Integration Dysfunction: A breakdown in the normal routing of sensory information. There may be difficulty in the perception, transmission, registration, or use of the senses in one's environment.

Sensory Hyposensitivity: A need for more than the normal amount of available sensory information in order for one to attend to, or to act upon, the environment.

Tactile Defensiveness: A negative reaction to touch, and/or avoidance or interaction with people or objects.

Oral Defensiveness: Tactile defensiveness of the mouth or cheek areas of the face.

Gravitational Insecurity: A negative reaction to changes in body position, especially when the feet are off the ground.

COMMUNICATION

Alluding to one's ability to speak or write (transmit), hear or read (receive), and understand messages.

Profoundly Delayed Language Abilities: Lack of age appropriate abilities to communicate (one year or more below one's actual age)

- *Receptive:* understanding words, symbols, gestures, etc.
- *Expressive:* use of written or spoken words, gestures, body language, etc.

SOCIO-EMOTIONAL

Behaviors characterized by difficulty in the development of social interaction skills (the ability to perceive, understand, and act).

- *Pervasive/Autistic Like Tendencies:* preoccupation with sameness in the environment, inability to participate in social activities, and aversion to social confrontation.
- *Co-existing Psychological Factors:* the possible presence of depression, schizophrenia, Alzheimer's Disease, etc.

Chapter 2
Structuring Programs and Activites

Those of us who work with people with profound developmental disabilities often wonder if group work is optimal for training/learning. Bourland, Jablonski and Lockhart (1988) compared the effects of instructing adults with severe and profound mental retardation in small group versus individual settings. Performance measures were: on-task behavior, instructional interaction, maladaptive behaviors, and percentage correct on the instructional task. Results indicated that overall, individual instruction had no clear advantages. This is consistent with findings from previous studies (Favell, Favell and McGimsey, 1978; Storm and Willis, 1978; Alberto, Jobes, Sizemore, and Doran, 1980). This would suggest that, considering staff and budgetary issues, most of us will be working with clients in small group settings. This chapter is intended to provide ideas for staff who are approaching group work with some trepidation due to lack of knowledge in group dynamics. (These ideas can be applied to people with any level of mental retardation.)

There is an art to working with a group of people, especially if the individuals have profound developmental disabilities. This is a unique situation because, for the most part, these individuals usually need constant prompts to attend and participate. The reality is that we often find ourselves working one-on-one in a room with a group of people. The end result is that we don't have a true group experience—we have individuals sitting around waiting to be the next one-on-one.

This brings us to the question—what is a true group experience? A group activity implies that a) there is organization and structure and b) that all members are participating in a common experience. It should not be assumed that caregivers or even therapists automatically know how to do this...for the most part, people are trained to do individual programs and to take data for these programs. There is a big difference, however, between focusing your energy on one person at a time and focusing your energy on four or five or fifteen people at a time. And that is the crux of the issue of group work—you must be aware of the needs of all individuals at the same time. A knowledge of group dynamics is not only useful but essential, for there are benefits that can be derived only from the group experience. These include:

- Creating and nurturing connections between individuals [interaction and socialization]

- Stimulating interplay and intercommunication both verbally and non-verbally [communication]

- Increasing sensitivity to peers and learning how to behave/interact appropriately

- Creating and nurturing friendships, sharing, learning to help others, and receiving emotional support

It is a challenge to work in a group setting. There will often be extenuating circumstances that impede the process; maladaptive behaviors, health problems, unrealistic demands for special attention, and real needs for special attention. It is always the responsibility of the staff person to keep the group together and focused, for the important unit is the group. There are individual goals we must work on, but there are also group goals. Group goals generally focus on the areas of socialization, interaction, and communication.

I. CREATING A GROUP

There are several important factors to consider when forming a group. These are

A. Membership:

Who will be in this group? Sometimes caregivers do not have a choice, but often it is possible to group people yourself. Groups should be as homogeneous as possible; that is, members should have some common bond. The bond could be physical ability, verbal ability, similar in favorite activities, similar training needs, etc. If possible, members should be chosen after the purpose of the group is established, not vice versa. The size of the group must also be considered in relation to the type of activity and the personalities involved.

B. Location:

Where will this group be? It is important to make sure that there is enough room for the activities you have planned—but it is also important to consider that the room might be too big. A large room can be a problem if you have individuals that are likely to wander or run. Other factors to consider are: how noisy is this environment?, how private is this room?, (will there be constant interruptions by people or telephones?), and is this room too hot, too cold, too dark, etc.?

C. Seating:

How will you organize this group? Where will the group leader sit in relation to everyone else? Sometimes we forget how important this is, for example, it is better to seat friends together and enemies apart. People who need extra assistance could be seated next to caregiver or to a peer who is able to, and enjoys, helping others. Most important—groups should be formed in a circle, or something closely resembling a circle. This is of major importance for several reasons:
- All members can see each other
- The group leader can see all the members
- All members become involved simply by being a part of the circle, even if they don't actively participate [inclusion]

The importance of the seating arrangement cannot be stressed enough. It is almost impossible to have a true group experience if people are all over the place. Creating a circle means creating organization, structure, unity, and inclusion.

D. Materials:

Do you have everything you need for a successful experience? If not, learn to be creative. Great activities really depend upon the attitude and creativity of the staff. For example, I once observed a music therapist creating a rhythm band using body sounds because there were no rhythm instruments available. I have observed a recreation therapist using a pillow for a game of catch because no ball was available (and the pillow was actually easier to throw and less intimidating than a ball). I know a recreation aide who saves everything because someday she will need it for a crafts activity. This woman always has materials!

II. WORKING WITH INDIVIDUALS IN GROUPS (PROCESSES)

A. Interaction and Inclusion:

Once people are seated in a circle, inclusion is a lot easier. The important points to remember are:

- **Encourage all members to listen or to watch the one person you are focusing on.** For example, if you have asked John a question, and he is taking some time to answer, ask some of the other group members questions such as "Are you listening? John is about to talk." or "Mark, could you repeat that question to John?". It is possible to do this in every situation with every type of individual. You can use physical prompts to encourage people to look at each other. This enables everyone to be part of the group experience.

- **Use people's names as often as possible.** Calling out someone's name usually gets their attention. Refer to people as much as you can—for example, if you are talking about the weather, point out that John is wearing warm clothes, Mark is not, etc. If you are singing songs, use individual names as often as possible. For example, in the song "He's Got The Whole World In His Hands", instead of singing "He's got you and me brother," try singing "He's got my friend John." You can do this with every group member, and it not only gets attention but also helps the members learn each other's names.

- **Encourage individuals to talk to each other, not just to staff.**
  If your group members are verbal, encourage them to ask each other questions. You do not always have to be the leader. It is much more natural for peers to interact among themselves.

B. Behavioral Issues

- **Minor Interruptions:** If possible, try to ignore these or redirect the individual back to the activity. Sometimes special attention paid to all the other group members will help.
- **Incidents of Inappropriate Behavior:** Usually there no is choice…if an inappropriate behavior occurs, caregivers have to intervene and this is a major interruption. Do the best you can, but try to return to the activity as soon as possible. Let the other group members know that they are important too, and praise them for their appropriate behavior!

C. Reinforcement

Reinforcement is very important. Caregivers must be certain they know what is really reinforcing to people. Giving everyone the same reinforcer may be easier, but in the long run it will not serve its purpose. Be consistent. Do not promise anything you can not deliver. Do let group members know when one person is being reinforced for good behavior. It is good for group members to know that positive reinforcement does exist and that they, too, can earn it.

D. Communication

Caregivers who are working with people with developmental disabilities must be constantly aware of communication issues. Generally our clients cannot process information at the speed or complexity with which most caregivers speak. This appears obvious, but it is easy to forget when one is working with a group of people. The following should be remembered at all times:

- **Directions should be simple and clear.**
  When one is training, too many cues can be confusing. Too much extra language can also be confusing. Examples:
  DO NOT: (pointing to water faucet) "Mark, why don't you try to grasp that handle and turn on the water so you can wash your hands and then we'll be able to go have dinner."
  DO: (pointing to faucet) "Mark, turn on the water please."
  DO NOT: "John, you can't hold the bell that way— it won't make any sound. You have to hold this end and keep your fingers off the bell part and then shake it."
  DO: "John, no. Try it this way" (and demonstrate).
- **Tone of voice should be calm and pleasant.** Caregivers should be aware of how they come across to other people. If your voice is naturally loud and your tone boisterous, you may have to work on bringing it down a notch. If you speak too softly, this can be very frustrating, especially if group members are hearing impaired. People everywhere respond to the way they are spoken to…respect earns respect, hostility usually creates hostility. The same is true for people with developmental disabilities. Sometimes caregivers cause inappropriate behavior because of inappropriate communication.

III. GROUP STRUCTURE AND ACTIVITIES

In most groups, if the leader is prepared and organized, the group will be more cohesive and organized. Activities should always be selected ahead of time, and these should relate to the individual and group goals. Materials should be out and ready. Most important—you should provide choices, be open to suggestions, and be ready to change and adapt at a moment's notice.

A. Starting and Concluding a Session

Always let your group know when the session is beginning and ending. It helps to define the time frame. In Music Therapy sessions, for example, the therapist starts with a "Hello" song and ends with a "Good-bye" song. This provides structure and it becomes a familiar signal to group members so they know what to expect.

B. Number of Activities

It is always effective to have a variety of activities, but you should try not to plan too many. One activity may be all that is needed (such as a game of BINGO) because it requires a lot of time. It is important to remember that activities may take longer with people with profound developmental disabilities, and they will probably need a lot of repetition. Often caregivers will feel that group members are becoming bored with an activity, although it is likely that the caregiver will become bored long before anyone else.

C. Types of Activities

Activities should be chosen to foster group experience. This appears obvious, but it does not always occur. Just because people are seated in a common area does not mean they are sharing an experience. The best activities for groups involve everyone at the same time (such as playing music, dancing, manipulating a parachute, etc.). If this is not possible, second best are activities that involve taking turns or teamwork (board games, horseshoes, Bingo, baseball, etc.). Group members can be encouraged to watch each other, cheer for each other, and assist each other. Activities that are not group oriented include watching TV (unless there is a group discussion about the show), arts and crafts (unless everyone is working together on a group project) and looking at magazines. These activities are more individualized. As stated above, group activities should involve everyone in a common task.

IV. PSYCHOLOGICAL ISSUES

Groups are important because they are good therapy! Peer interaction can be supportive and can help increase and develop good self esteem. Most of the time it is more fun to participate in activities with other people so that experiences can be shared. Groups help people learn to get along with others, to communicate, to take turns, to develop responsibility, and to work with others toward a common goal. In other words, groups can help people learn life skills.

In conclusion, the importance of groups cannot be stressed enough, even with individuals with profound disabilities who do not appear to be cognizant of others. Gardner and Chapman (1991) state that

"The design and evaluation of program plans focus on the individual for most identified objectives, however, the implementation of program plans takes place within a group.

The focus of instruction is on individual objectives within group settings and activities. Active treatment is measured by the effectiveness of the instructors' (mostly the direct care staff) ability to implement effectively individualized objectives in a group setting, as defined by the measurable outcomes in client growth and development." (p. 100)

All of us belong to groups in our daily lives: work, religious affiliations, community activities, and family. We turn to group members for support, intellectual stimulation, fun, love, shared interests, shared problems, and companionship. People with developmental disabilities have these same needs, and these can be met most effectively through opportunities to participate in meaningful group experiences.

Chapter 3
Considerations for Functional Communication

Professional attention toward the needs of people with developmental disabilities has risen in recent years. Research specifically regarding communication with individuals with profound mental retardation has received relatively little attention when it is compared to research on communication with other populations. In past years, such individuals were considered uncommunicative and received very little attention and even less intervention. However, in recent years, many gains addressing behavioral and communicative challenges have been made. This section will address the notion of communicative competence as it relates to people with developmental disabilities. Particular attention will be given to the utilization of nonverbal communication, more commonly referred to as body language. Suggestions will be provided as to how caregivers may improve their knowledge of an individual's communicative behavior through the compilation of communication dictionaries and influenced through the use of communication scenarios.

COMMUNICATION, LANGUAGE, AND SPEECH

Before considering the concept of communication with individuals with profound mental retardation, one must first consider exactly what makes up communication. Then, one must understand the nature of both speech and language; and, more importantly, how these three concepts are related. This chapter will address these subjects, and, upon an explanation of each, attention will be given to how they are perceived with individuals with developmental disabilities.

First, *communication is the exchange of ideas and concepts*. When one talks on the telephone, one communicates. When a person sends a memo, he communicates. When a person gives another person a nasty look, he communicates. Communication is both an active and a passive process. Actively; we gossip, we send birthday cards, we write books, etc. Passively, in order to communicate, we may wear a particular outfit to an event or function, we may sit at particular positions in a board meeting, etc. It is a common misconception that people with profound mental retardation do not actively communicate; however, these individuals, more often than not, make their needs known through behavior. These behaviors may come in the form of vocalizations, or they could occur as self-injurious behaviors (hitting/biting themselves, etc.).

Second, language refers to *any rule-governed system of communication*. Language may be spoken or written (e.g. English, French, etc.). They may even be gestural (involving movements of the body) as with sign language or generated through a computer's electrical impulses. (Computer languages are made up of "binary" codes—series and combinations of 1 and 0 which represent different letters or commands.) In fact, there are literally tens of thousands of languages in use today, and several more that are now extinct. Languages, like cities and people, are constantly changing and evolving. With respect to people with profound mental retardation, DSM-IV states that these individuals achieve a developmental language age equivalent of one to two years. Developmentally, the period between one and two years is the prime time for which the roots of language development are formed. During that period, individuals learn that words have meaning and using words makes things happen.

Speech (oral motor or movement of the mouth and its structures) is simply ONE *means by which an individual accesses a language in order to communicate.* If a person is deaf, he may use various configurations of his hands to access sign language. He can then communicate with a hearing-impaired peer. When a person writes or types, he puts pen to paper or fingers to keyboard to access letters to form words and sentences. In consideration of people with profound mental retardation, such individuals seldom develop usable speech, and, thus, they are unable to access their home language in that manner. They often suffer from more severe physical limitations by which they are unable to access sign language or sophisticated computers.

COMMUNICATIVE COMPETENCE

As previously stated, individuals with profound mental retardation often use socially inappropriate behavior as their main method of communication. These behaviors may be both active or passive. The particular behavior may be reflexive or purposeful in that the individual is using the behavior to avoid an undesirable action. The behavior also may be used to indicate a request. The behavior may be a sign of frustration as a result of a request not being answered or a need not addressed. Or, the behavior may be a nonfunctional habit learned over time. Regardless of the motivation behind the communicative behavior, the most important concept to understand is how USEFUL the behavior is in getting the individual's point across. Whether or not an individual's needs are met after the communicative behavior is an indication of his/her communicative competence.

As stated earlier, communication can be considered as simply getting from point A to point B. The success or ease by which any individual is able to travel between these two points can be termed as communicative competence. Thus, communicative competence may be considered as how well an individual is able to transmit a message (or concept or idea, etc.) *And* how well it can be received (if at all). Using this definition, many people figure that

people with mental retardation are somewhat incompetent when it comes to communication. However, this population, through trial and error, has become very adept in this perspective.

It is important to note that we are all subject to communicative competence. For example, let's say that you have to give a speech. You prepared your presentation for months and are finally ready to give it. Right before you start, you find out that your entire audience is from a foreign country, and you do not speak that language. In that regard, you are communicatively incompetent. That is an extreme example; however, there are infinite cultural, gender, educational, class, and/or regional differences between individuals that serve directly to inhibit anyone's ability to communicate effectively (Tannen, 1990). This is increased when individuals remain insensitive to these differences. Thus, it is important to note that all individuals communicate in some fashion, both actively and passively, both purposefully (with a specific goal in mind) AND reflexively (as a result of certain stimuli). It is the job of all of us to accept that these differences exist. And *more importantly,* it is our job to look beyond the differences and seek the motivating factors behind the "communicative behavior."

VERBAL VERSUS NONVERBAL COMMUNICATION

It was previously stated that communication is both active and passive. Communication or communicative behaviors are also *verbal* (involving the use of words, speech, and/or symbols) and *nonverbal*. Nonverbal communication includes gestures (including fine and gross body movements, facial movements, eye behaviors, and postures). (Beukelman and Mirenda, 1992). Nonverbal behaviors may also include other more specific types of body posture, i.e., objectics, kinesics, proxemics, optics, and chronemics. (These will be defined in the next section.) Nonverbal behaviors may also be prosodic (vocal characteristics dependent upon mood and situation). Prosodic features include pitch (how high or low a sound may be), intonation (accent or stress on a word or part of a word), stress, and volume (the loudness or softness of a sound). As people with profound mental retardation seldom learn usable speech, their communicative behaviors may be classified as primarily nonverbal.

MARKERS FOR NONVERBAL COMMUNICATION

It is interesting to consider that we are able to understand a person's wants, needs, feelings, and/or ideas without the other person uttering a single word. When we are able to read someone's mood, we are first utilizing that individual's nonverbal behaviors and, second, lending meaning to the behaviors based on our own experiences. When we realize that someone is in an agitated mood, we often avoid that person or give them some space. We can often tell that something is wrong by the way they dress (he/she may have been a meticulous dresser and is now messy). We can sense that they are in a foul mood by the way in which they carry themselves (they may have previously been a very upbeat and animated person and now they are acting cold towards us). These are just two examples of how people receive a nonverbal message. By first receiving the message, we can then appropriately interact with that individual by providing support or comfort (if needed) or no interaction at all (if appropriate). This same process is useful when attempting to communicate with people with developmental disabilities. By careful and extensive observation, we can accurately chart specific behaviors exhibited by our clients and then apply meaning to each of the behaviors observed. This is the basic process by which professionals often compile (our previously mentioned) communication or gestural dictionaries. However, prior to presenting a method for dictionary compilation, one must first view a listing of specific types of nonverbal behaviors:

Objectics: Use of objects (clothes, utensils, etc.)
Example: A client shows you a cup to ask for more to drink.

Kinesics: Movement of a specific body part to enhance communication
Example: A client may shake his/her hand in the air to gain attention.

Proxemics: Use of barriers and whole body placement to enhance communication
Example: A client moves away as a particular staff member approaches.

Optics: Involving eye moments
Example: A client may avert his/her gaze from a person or task in order to say no or avoid a particular situation or job.

Chronemics: Involving the timing and spacing of words and actions in order to enhance a message
Example: A client may increase or decrease his/her rate of action or speech in order to protest an action or delay an undesired duty.

THE COMMUNICATION DICTIONARY

As stated previously, the communication dictionary is very useful in providing the caregiver with knowledge about how an individual communicates. The process of compiling a communication dictionary can entail varying degrees of difficulty. Some behaviors may be easy to code and add to a list and others will require persistent observation over a long time period. We all have certain unique behaviors which clearly stand out to others and have other behaviors which are completely unseen unless someone is closely observed (e.g., a person always sitting in a particular place at a weekly meeting, or even tapping his/her fingers on a desk when deep in thought). It is important to note that such a process can aid both the caregiver and those unfamiliar with an individual in interpreting some behaviors. It can also help to de-escalate some maladaptive behaviors because as one becomes more aware of how a client communicates, one is better able to predict and react more appropriately to a certain behavior. The caregiver can then react to the behavior more quickly and appropriately. The following is one simple example of how a communication dictionary can be compiled.

The communication dictionary is just the beginning of proactive communication strategies with this population. It helps in a variety of ways; but more importantly, it may ease some caregiver's hesitation or reluctance in working with these people. It proves beneficial to use the communication dictionary as a starting point. As caregivers become more adept at identifying communicative behaviors, they may begin to utilize the time periods of occurrence to teach clients more advanced communicative tasks, e.g., 1) using social greetings, 2) asking for help, and/or 3) using a functional yes/no response.

It is our sincere hope that caregivers will utilize the communication dictionary as an integral part of all scenarios. By being able to identify or predict communicative behaviors, caregivers can utilize the scenarios better thus increasing the likelihood for success.

COMMUNICATION DICTIONARY

SAMPLE OBSERVABLE BEHAVIORS:

Facial Expressions:
Smiling
Frowning
Grimacing
Twitching

Eye Movements:
Blinking
Gazing
Gaze aversion
Staring
Widening eyes
Closing eyes
Tracking

Head Movements:
Nodding
Shaking head from
  side to side
Throwing head back
Raising head
Lowering head

Gross Motor Movements:
Running away
Swiping
Flailing arms
Stamping feet
Turning away
Turning toward
Rolling

Clapping
Banging
Kicking
Rocking
Reaching
Crawling
Jumping

Postural Changes:
Flopping
Fixing in reflex patterns
  i.e. _____
Tensing
Localizing to visual input
Localizing to sound
Changing muscle tone

Actions on Objects:
Banging
Mouthing
Throwing
Biting
Bringing to ears
Bringing to eyes

Smelling
Pushing
Pulling
Shaking
Spinning
Stroking

Vocalizations:
Crying
Producing vowel
  sounds
Producing consonant
  sounds
Clucking tongue

Moaning
Screaming
Gurgling
Singing
Cooing
Grunting

Manual Gestures:
Pointing
Tapping
Grasping
Raising hand
Touching
Grabbing
Waving
Pushing
Pulling
Manual signs or approximations

Oral-Motor Movements:
Opening mouth
Closing mouth
Sticking out tongue
Puckering lips

ASHA Convention 1995, Poster Session #1081
Presenter: Jane G. Shulman, M.S., CCC-SLP
               182-36 80th Drive
               Jamaica, N.Y. 11432 (718) 380-6308

COMMUNICATION DICTIONARY
INFORMATION-GATHERING FORM

Client's Name:_____ Date:_____

Therapist's Name:_____

PART I. How Do I Communicate?

I _____ to say I'm happy. These things make me happy:

_____

I _____ to say I'm unhappy. These things make me unhappy:

_____

I _____ to say I'm hungry.

I _____ to say I'm thirsty

I _____ to say I'm wet.

I _____ to say I'm tired/bored.

I _____ to say I'm in pain/uncomfortable.

I _____ to say "Yes."

I _____ to say "No."

I _____ to choose or show preference.

I _____ to request attention.

I _____ to request desired objects or activities.

I _____ to reject.

Other important information:_____

_____

ASHA Convention 1995, Poster Session #1081
Presenter: Jane G. Shulman, M.S., CCC-SLP
              182-36 80th Drive
              Jamaica, N.Y. 11432 (718) 380-6308

PART TWO

The Scenarios

Chapter 4

Introduction and Important Considerations for the Scenarios

INTRODUCTION:

The Scenarios are grouped together into seven categories for easy reference. These groupings identify the major focus of the activities, but many address multiple categories:

- **Activities of Daily Living:**
  Activities related to self-care, homemaking, and all general daily needs.

- **Sensory Stimulation:**
  Activities related to all the senses.

- **Gross Motor:**
  Activities related to broad body movement, particularly the torso, arms and legs.

- **Fine Motor:**
  Activities related to smaller body movements, particularly hands and fingers.

- **Cognitive:**
  Activities related to functional interaction, choice making and self-advocacy.

- **Communication:**
  Activities related to attending, cause and effect, and aumentative and alternative methods of communication.

- **Social/Recreation:**
  Activities related to social interaction, leisure, and artistic expression.

Each scenario is presented in the same format: Purpose (Goals), Materials, Preferred Setting, Procedure, and Reminders (if applicable). All materials listed for each scenario that need to be made by hand or purchased are referenced in Part 3.

IMPORTANT

In the process of collaborating on the scenarios, we found that several points surfaced consistently over and over again. We offer these as important considerations for the effective implementation of any scenario:

Prompting: Levels of Assistance

Allow for the least amount of assistance at the beginning of each activity. Assume that the client is independent and then if they do need help, work backwards from the least amount of help to the most:

- **Verbal prompt:**
  (Speaking without touching)
- **Gestural prompt:**
  (Pointing without touching)
- **Tactile prompt:**
  (Touching or tapping the client and/or the object)
- **Faded physical prompt:**
  (Hand-over-hand assistance to begin with, which is slowly removed)
- **Physical prompt:**
  (Hand-over-hand assistance)

Following this procedure, the client always has the maximum opportunity to be as independent as possible. Often caregivers assume that people with profound mental retardation cannot complete tasks because of their development level. However, we've found that if given ample opportunity, our clients often surprise us with their own ingenuity and inventiveness.

Communication: Talking To Clients

Talk to adults with profound mental retardation the same way you talk to other adults. Though they may have difficulty with receptive language, they still deserve the opportunity to listen and understand, and perhaps they *may* understand something you've said. Often the only verbalizations addressed to them are directives, reprimands and greetings, in that order. Everyone deserves the opportunity to hear adult topics of conversation; talk to clients about your families, feelings, the environment, the daily news, etc. Include clients in your conversations with co-workers, friends and family. They may not understand the context of the discussion but they may feel a sense of inclusion.

Socialization: Utilizing Opportunities

Always encourage interaction and socialization at every opportunity. Adults with profound mental retardation often live in social isolation, unaware of the people and possibilities around then. Encouraging clients to look at, interact with, and listen to each other is one step toward expanding their world.

Adaptations: Knowledge of Client Needs

Consider the special needs of each person when you are planning activities. If unsure, consult with the therapist, physician, nurse, psychologist, or any professional person who might have the expertise you need. The scenarios will be most beneficial if adapted to meet the individual's needs.

Safety: Knowledge of Client Behaviors

Be aware of any maladaptive behaviors which could be safety risk. For example, a client may have Pica (eating loose environmental objects). Many of the scenarios utilize small objects which could be easily ingested causing a host of medical problems.

Inclusion: Creating Opportunities

It is of the utmost importance that you include people with profound mental retardation in all aspects of daily living. The scenarios provide structured ideas, but the point is that there are opportunities for learning in every situation. If you provide opportunities, and assume that abilities do exist, it is likely you will discover some abilities. This is a difficult endeavor, especially if you have a *group* of clients at all times. Remember that it is important to celebrate the small steps—turning to look at you, attending to your voice, grasping an object. Any time you create an opportunity, you increase the likelihood for positive change. And it is through positive change that all individuals learn and grow.

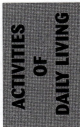

CHAPTER 5

Activities of Daily Living

1. Music Assisted Personal Grooming
2. Skin Care
3. Hair Care
4. Pre-Dressing Skills
5. Adaptive Fastener Frames
6. Meal Preparation
7. Beverage Preparation
8. Homemaking
9. Using Switches

Music-Assisted Personal Grooming

Purpose:
• Increase independence in self-help skills
• Develop/increase skills in following simple directions
• Develop cues to learn a skill sequence
• Provide motivation for completing a task

Materials:
• Regular items used for bathing, brushing teeth, etc.

Preferred Setting:
This activity should take place in the natural setting where self-care would occur.

Procedure:
This activity requires the caregiver to sing using a simple song, written with the intent of motivating the client to participate actively in the self care task. The following are suggestions for songs that can be used:

1. *To the tune of "Do Lord"*
   Wanda, oh Wanda, oh Wanda wash your face (neck, back, etc.)
   Wanda, oh Wanda, oh Wanda wash your face
   Wanda, oh Wanda, oh Wanda wash your face
   Wash your face right now.

2. *To the tune of "Kumbaya"*
   Sandy brush your teeth, brush them now
   Sandy brush your teeth, brush them now
   Brush the teeth on top (bottom), brush them now
   Oh, Sandy, brush your teeth.

3. *To the tune of "Old Brass Wagon"*
   Comb your hair, my friend Richard
   Comb your hair, my friend Richard
   Comb your hair, my friend Richard
   Comb your hair this morning.

Reminders:
1. Make sure songs are age-appropriate. With these types of activities there is a tendency to remember children's songs and use them.
2. If you can come up with an effective rap-type chant, use it! Sometimes rhythm works just as well as melody.

Skin Care

Purpose:
- To increase participation in grooming tasks
- To increase functional motion of arms and hands required for grooming activities
- To increase awareness of body parts
- To increase exposure to a variety of tactile and olfactory sensory materials

Materials:
- Skin lotion
- Perfume(for women)
- Aftershave (for men)

Preferred Setting:
Tabletop, or the natural setting where this type of grooming activity occurs as part of the daily routine, such as the bedroom or bathroom.

Procedure:
1. Encourage clients to apply the skin lotion, perfume, or after shave to their hands and/or arms. Clients should have the opportunity to do this as independently as possible, with physical assistance given only when needed.
2. Encourage the individual to smell the cosmetic before application (from the container) and after application (on the hands or arms).
3. Encourge peer awareness by instructing clients to apply the cosmetic to the hands of another group member.

Reminders:
1. Refer to the Scenario titled "Music-Assisted Personal Grooming." The same principles can be applied here.
2. Encourage as much independence as possible. Consider that the client is capable of completing at least one small part of the total task.

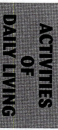

Hair Care

Purpose:
- To increase participation in self-help activities
- To improve functional movements of arms and hands
- To provide visual and tactile sensory stimulation
- To encourage bilateral use of arms
- To increase body awareness

Materials:
- Items related to the particular task: washing, drying, combing and styling hair. See Part 3 for ideas regarding adaptive equipment for people with physical limitations.
- Mirror (hand held, tabletop or wall mounted) should be available for visual feedback.

Preferred Setting:
It would be most appropriate to work on hair care in the setting where this activity would naturally occur (bedroom or bathroom).

Procedure:
1. Place the materials for hair care on the counter in front of the clients. As you move through the various phases of each task, encourage the clients to participate as fully as possible, even if they are only capable of completing a small portion of the entire task. For example:
   a. Picking up the comb or brush
   b. Selecting a barrette from a box of choices
   c. Holding up the mirror (for self or someone else)
   d. Partially raising up the towel for hair drying
   e. Pouring shampoo onto the hand
2. If the activity is done in a group and is more focused on setting and/or styling hair, encourage the clients to look at each other as this is occurring. Ensure that each person has the opportunity to see themselves in the mirror.
3. Talk about each phase of the task as it occurs.

Reminders:
1. Refer to the Scenario titled "Music-Assisted Personal Grooming." The same principles can be applied here.
2. Encourage as much independence as possible. Consider that the client is capable of completing at least one small part of the total task.

Pre-Dressing Skills

Purpose:
- To increase participation in dressing tasks
- To increase functional arm and hand skills required for dressing activities
- To increase awareness of body parts
- To increase exposure to a variety of tactile and visual sensory materials

Materials:
- Mirror (provides visual feedback and reinforces cause and effect)
- Predressing Kit (consisting of hats, scarves, neckties, bracelets, necklaces)

Preferred Setting:
Tabletop with portable mirror, or within close proximity of a wall-mounted mirror. If possible, this activity should be done in the environment in which dressing normally occurs, such as the bedroom or bathroom.

Procedure:
1. Ask the client to sit in front of the mirror or place the client in front of the mirror if he/she is not able to follow this verbal request.
2. Ask the client to select a desired item from the box (Predressing Kit). Provide the opportunity for the client to do this independently and provide assistance only as needed.
3. Select an item for yourself, and encourage the clients to watch you as you demonstrate how to put on the item (e.g., "John, look at me. I'm putting the hat on my head.")
4. Ask the client to do what you just did ("Now it's your turn, John. Put the hat on your head.") Encourage the client to do this independently and offer assistance only as needed.
5. After the client is wearing the item, provide a verbal cue to look in the mirror. ("John, look at how nice the hat looks on your head.") Encourage group members to look at each other. ("Wayne, look at how great John looks in that hat.")
6. After each client is wearing an item from the box and discussion has ensued, work on the process of taking the items off. As before, cue each person to look at themselves in the mirror, and to watch their peers.

Reminders:
1. The use of the mirror is important. Many individuals do not have enough opportunities to see what they look like, and to see themselves engaged in different activities.
2. Remember to use gender appropriate items, and to include any items in your Kit that might be special for a certain person. The predressing kit can consist of any additional items you would like to add, but it is recommended that you begin by working with small items used around the head or neck.
3. Encourage choices!

Adaptive Fastener Frames

Purpose:
- To increase ability to manipulate clothing fasteners
- To increase fine motor coordination
- To increase visual attention to task
- To increase exposure to a variety of tactile and visual sensory materials

Materials:
- Fastener Frames (See Part 3 for resources and for ideas on how to make your own.)

Preferred Setting:
Tabletop

Procedure:
1. Ask the client to choose a fastener frame with which he/she would like to work. Encourage the client to make a choice if he/she is not able to respond to the question. Look for cues, such as turning of the head toward a particular frame.
2. Verbally cue the client to watch you as you demonstrate how to work the fastener (e.g., "Judy, this is how you close the velcro." or "Watch me work the zipper, Robert.")
3. Encourage the client to work the fastener, always allowing for as much independence as possible. Offer assistance only if needed. Verbally cue the client to watch their hands as they work on the task.
4. It would also be beneficial to have the individual practice the manipulation of similar clothing fasteners on their own clothes. This should only be done after practice with the fastener frames.
5. Talk to the individual about the type of fastener with which they are working. Ask them to locate that type of fastener on their clothes or on the clothes of other members of the group.
6. If clients are experiencing difficulty with this task, increase their sensory awareness of the materials. For example, encourage them to visually attend to the color or pattern of the fabric. Ensure that they touch and manipulate the various textures.

Reminders:
1. Encourage group interaction whenever possible.
2. Be aware of hand dominance for each individual and encourage use of the preferred hand for these tasks.

Meal Preparation

Purpose:
- To encourage active participation in daily living activities
- To encourage functional movement of arms
- To improve eye-hand coordination
- To provide an opportunity to assume a caregiver role
- To develop the ability to follow directions
- To develop sequencing skills
- To reinforce basic spatial concepts (on/off, in/out, beside, etc.)

Materials:
- Items related to the particular meal preparation task. (See Part 3 for ideas regarding adaptive equipment for people with physical limitations.)

Preferred Setting:
These activities must be carried out in their natural setting (kitchen and/or dining room).

Procedure:
1. Encourage clients to retrieve materials for the particular meal preparation task.
2. As you move through the steps of the task, encourage clients to perform independently as much of the task as possible, if the total task is too difficult. For example:
   a. Operate a switch to turn on an appliance.
   b. Pour a measured item into a bowl.
   c. Pick up a wooden spoon and hand it to the caregiver or a peer.
   d. Pull open a cabinet door.
   e. Shake salt or pepper over a designated area.
   f. Stir or mix ingredients in a bowl.
   g. Wash vegetables by holding a collander under running water.
   h. Fold a napkin.
   i. Place flatware in designated places on a placemat.
3. Each of the tasks listed above, or others, can be pared down to even simpler components. For example, if the client is unable to fold a napkin, perhaps he or she can hold down one edge while you fold it. Or, if the client is unable to stir ingredients, perhaps he or she could hold both sides of the bowl while you stir.

Reminders:
1. Be aware of allergies and diet restrictions of all group members.
2. Encourage group interaction as much as possible. Some tasks may be able to be done in assembly line fashion which would encourage taking turns.

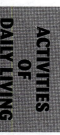

Beverage Preparation

Purpose:
- To increase independence with and participation in meal preparation tasks
- To improve gross motor motions of upper extremities
- To increase bilateral use of arms
- To encourage socialization skills

Materials:
- Pitcher
- Cups, glasses, spoon (utilize adaptive cup or utensil if needed due to physical limitations)
- Powdered drink mix

Preferred Setting:
Structure or schedule the group in an environment that meal preparation and the consumption of food initially takes place (near a sink or at a countertop). Once preparation of liquid is completed, the group can be relocated to a table for pouring and drinking of the beverage. This will increase the opportunities for socialization among group members.

Procedure:
1. Encourage clients to retrieve needed supplies from the storage area.
2. As the group facilitator, you may want to assign each client a particular job or ask for a volunteer for each step:
   a. turn on water faucet;
   b. fill pitcher with water;
   c. add powdered mix to water;
   d. stir liquid with spoon until particles are dissolved.
   (This step is appropriate for participation by all clients through taking turns.)
3. Clients can be encouraged to pour their own glass of liquid or one group member can serve the others.
4. Encourage socialization as much as possible during this activity, particularly when they are drinking the beverage. For example:
   a. Encourage clients to hand cups to one another.
   b. Encourage eye contact through verbal cue, tactile cues, or physical assistance.
   c. Encourage clients to communicate vocally, through body language, or by pointing. (Caregivers can also communicate with clients using these alternative methods.)
   d. Ask clients "yes/no" questions. (They are easier to understand than open-ended questions)

Reminders:
1. Be aware of allergies and diet restrictions of all group members.
2. Use appropriate background music to add to the social aspect of the activity (probably sedative-type music would be most appropriate).
3. Encourage choices whenever possible (e.g., the cup the client will use or the flavor of beverages if you have more than one).

Homemaking

Procedure:

For the purposes of this scenario, cleaning/dusting will be the task described. The principles can be applied to other tasks such as washing dishes, doing laundry, etc.:

1. Explain the cleaning/dusting task to the client, and, if possible, encourage the client to choose a piece of furniture to dust.
2. Show the client the dusting cloth and the polish and give the client the opportunity to touch and feel the texture of the cloth and to smell the polish. Explain that these are the items used for dusting and demonstrate their use.
3. Encourage the client to spray the polish on the piece of furniture, providing assistance as needed.
4. Encourage the client to rub the polish onto the furniture, providing physical assistance only if necessary. If this task is done in a group, encourage the other group members to watch until it is their turn. Depending upon the task, you can also assign different parts of each task to different group members.

Reminders:

1. Encourage independence as much as possible. Take every opportunity to teach skills and break these skills down to their simplest parts if necessary.
2. If you would like to use background music to create a pleasant environment for working, it might be best to choose music that is more stimulative in nature. Often music provides the stimulation necessary to encourage movement, so music that is rhythmic and upbeat would be of benefit.

Purpose:
- To encourage active participation in daily living activities
- To improve functional movement of arms
- To improve eye-hand coordination
- To provide an opportunity to assume a caregiver role
- To develop the ability to follow directions
- To develop sequencing skills
- To encourage mobility around environmental obstacles

Materials:
- Items related to the particular task (cleaning, dusting, stacking, etc.) (See Part 3 for ideas regarding adaptive equipment for people with physical limitations)

Preferred Setting:
These activities must be carried out in their natural setting.

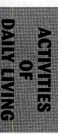

Using Switches

Purpose:
- To provide an alternate means for the activation of battery-operated or electrically-powered appliances
- To help establish/develop/reinforce knowledge of cause and effect

Materials:
- A simple pressure switch is easiest (See Part 3 for resources)
- Battery interrupter (See Part 3)
- Battery-operated household items, such as radios, tape recorders, etc.
- If possible to purchase, AbleNet@ "Powerlink" is a useful device, in that it allows individuals to activate larger electrically-powered items: mirrored lights, blenders, etc. (See Part 3 for resources)

Preferred Setting:
This scenario is best performed one-on-one in a quiet environment

Procedure:
1. Place the individual's hand on the switch (if client is physically able to use hands). (Encourage use of other body parts if hands are nonfunctional, such as arms, knees, etc.)
2. Gain the individual's attention (or place item directly in the individual's focus).
3. Using hand-over-hand (hand-over-body part) assistance, lightly press down on the switch for activation.
4. Reinforce the procedure verbally to the individual.
5. Lightly remove the individual's hand/body part from the switch, to cease activation.
6. Repeat steps two through five.

Reminders:
1. Ensure that the switch is activating an item that is meaningful to the individual.
2. If activating something that plays music, remember that music influences behavior, so choose music according to preference and mood.
3. There are many different types of switches, that can be activated in non-traditional ways (such as by a puff of breath, a tilt of the head, etc.). Many catalogs listed in Part 3 offer these alternatives.

CHAPTER 6

Sensory Stimulation

1. Aromas

2. Nature Box

3. Dark Box/Column

4. Find the Musical Sound

5. Find the Sound

6. Music—Playing Rhythm Instruments

7. Music and Tactile Defensiveness

8. Vibration

9. Texture Rub

10. Brushing

11. Deep Massage

12. Water Exploration

13. Sponges

14. Walking

Aromas

Purpose:
- To increase level of arousal
- To provide olfactory (smell) stimulation
- To encourage socialization with caregivers

Materials:
- Aroma Kit—available commercially through specialized catalogs. (See Part 3 for resources.) This kit can be easily made by collecting or purchasing various cooking extracts, spices, perfumes, etc. You could also use potpourri.
- Cotton balls

Preferred Setting:
This activity can occur anywhere, but preferably not in a location that has interfering scents.

Procedure:
1. Explain the activity to the individual.
2. Place a generous amount of one scent on a cotton ball.
3. Wave the cotton ball approximately three inches under the individual's nose for five seconds, making sure not to touch the person's nose.
4. Talk to the individual about what they are smelling. You may also want to show a picture of an object or the actual object that relates to this aroma (e.g., a perfume bottle, a picture of a pine tree, an orange, a picture of a rose).

Reminders:
An aroma can linger for a long time. Introducing one aroma immediately after another is usually ineffective. Present one aroma to each group member, then try the next.

Nature Box

Purpose:
- To increase functional motions of arms and hands
- To expose the client to a variety of visual, tactile, and olfactory stimuli
- To encourage socialization
- To increase orientation to and awareness of outdoor environment

Materials:
- Nature Box (collection of rocks, sea shells, pine cones, leaves, bark, artificial flowers, etc.)

Preferred Setting:
Tabletop, or outside environment if you would like to include the collecting of the nature items into the rest of the activity.

Procedure:
1. Begin by showing the client each item in the Nature Box. Encourage visual tracking of the item. If appropriate, touch the client's face or hand with the object.
2. Talk to the client about the object—it's size, shape, color, texture, scent. Talk about where in nature it is found.
3. Ask the client if he/she would like to hold the object. Give them the opportunity to reach/grasp the object independently. Offer assistance only as needed.
4. For individuals with limited motor abilities, you may have to take the item from the Nature Box and place it in their hands. Move the item around in the client's hands so they can feel it's size, shape and texture.
5. Encourage the client to manipulate one object for at least two minutes. During this time, talk to the client about the object they are holding.
6. Encourage the client to hand the object to another client in the group.
7. Allow ample opportunity for the exploration of numerous objects.

Reminders:
1. Be cautious of individuals placing objects in their mouth.
2. To enhance this activity, you can purchase and play tapes of nature sounds. You can also make your own tapes by recording sounds related to your activity.

Dark Box/ Column

Purpose:
- To provide a variety of visual and/or tactile sensory stimulation
- To improve functional motions of arms and hands
- To encourage socialization

Materials:
- See Resource Part 3 for instructions/ recommendations on how to construct the Dark Box/Column
- Flashlights
- Fluorescent paper and fluorescent mobiles

Preferred Setting:
Inside the Dark Box or Column (this will be explained in the Procedure section.)

Procedure:
The Dark Box/Column is an easily built structure that does not allow any light inside. This activity will make use of the lack of visual distractions to encourage clients to focus on specific tasks.

1. You may want to prepare the individual for placement in the dark box/column by turning off the lights in the room.
2. After placing the individual in the dark box/column, you can encourage attention to the environment and visual tracking by doing any of the following:
   a. Move the flashlight across the wall in the box/column
   b. Turn the flashlight on and off in rapid or random patterns
   c. Place fluorescent paper shapes or stringed lights on the wall. Use the flashlight to trace these different shapes.
   d. Move the fluorescent paper shapes through the environment with your hands.
   e. Use a small fan to create motion of the fluorescent paper mobiles hanging in the box.
3. Encourage the individuals to participate actively by holding and moving the flashlight, manipulating the fluorescent shapes, etc. If this is not possible, simply encourage individuals to look and track.

Reminders:
1. The Dark Box/Column needs to be large enough for two people: the client and the caregiver.
2. Ensure that the environment outside the box is not distracting (noisy). You can play sedative-type instrumental music to create a calm environment and help the client focus.

Find the Musical Sound

Purpose:
- Evoke a greater response to a sound stimulus.
- Develop responsiveness to the surrounding environment.

Materials:
- Several musical instruments with different sounds: bell, tambourine, egg shaker, chimes, etc.

Preferred Setting:
The only requirement for this setting is a quiet room, or a place that is quiet enough for the individual to locate the source of the sound you are making. This activity will need to be one-on-one.

Procedure:
This is an activity that is very simple to do. It is the first stage in developing auditory awareness or perhaps any kind of awareness of something in the environment.

The caregiver should stand behind the client and play an instrument near the client's ear (shake a bell, tambourine, etc.) Hopefully, the client will turn his/her head toward the source of the sound. This should be repeated near the other ear, over the client's head, and in any other direction that might be possible for client head movement. You do not want to do this where the client can see the instrument because this is not a visual task. Once the client has responded to the direction of the sound, you may give him/her the instrument to touch, play, or look at.

Reminders:
1. Do not play the instruments too loud—you do not want to scare the client, especially if you are right near the ear.
2. This activity can be done with items other than musical instruments, if they make an interesting noise, such as an alarm clock, a buzzer, or a whistle. Any environmental sounds are great to use because it increases the client's awareness of items they might find in a house or workshop.
3. Always be aware of client preferences when you are doing this activity. It might be a great time to find out what motivates the person to turn his/her head.

Find the Sound

Purpose:
• To increase environmental awareness
• To increase individuals' ability to track items in their environment by ear
• To enhance individuals' exposure to cause and effect

Materials:
• One large scarf or towel
• A tape recorder with a variety of environmental sounds (you can record these yourself)

Preferred Setting:
This scenario is best performed one-on-one in a quiet environment.

Procedure:
1. Place the recorder on a table directly in front of the individual.
2. Prompt the individual to focus on the tape recorder.
3. Press play to start the tape.
4. If the individual does not focus on the tape recorder, prompt the individual to look at the recorder.
5. Stop the tape.
6. Cover the tape recorder with the scarf.
7. Press play again.
8. If the individual does not focus attention on the sound source (the tape recorder), prompt his/her to focus on the scarf (where the sound comes from).
9. Repeat steps two through eight (placing the tape recorder at different positions around the table).

Procedure:
This activity can be done with other environmental items, such as an alarm clock, a buzzer or a telephone. The only requirement is that this item makes a sound on its own, so the client is not visually focusing on your hands.

Music— Playing Rhythm Instruments

Purpose:
- Increase exposure to a variety of auditory, tactile, visual (sensory) stimuli
- Increase involvement and participation in a musical activity
- Provide immediate sense of accomplishment and success
- Increase social interaction
- Improve attending behavior (and re-direct maladaptive behaviors)
- Reinforce cause-and-effect concept

Materials:
- Box of rhythm instruments. A wide assortment is recommended; many instruments can be made, if you prefer to do that. Part 3 provides ideas and instructions.
- Tape/CD Player with a variety of music that has a strong, steady beat.

Preferred Setting:
Large circle with enough room between people for caregivers to move in and out of the circle and around clients. (Individuals can then be assisted from behind and from their sides, so their view is not blocked.)

Procedure:
1. Take the box of instruments to each individual, encouraging choice. If necessary, narrow the choice by holding up two instruments. Encourage the client to stretch by reaching for the instrument of choice.
2. Designate one individual to assist with operating the tape/CD player, and assist them with this task throughout the activity (i.e., opening the player, placing the tape inside, and pressing the "on" switch). If necessary, use a switch-operated tape/CD player.
3. Throughout the song, assist the clients in playing the instruments, always encouraging independence first. Try the following variations while using the instruments:
   a. Encourage clients to play soft or loud.
   b. Encourage clients to play fast or slow.
   c. Encourage clients to play instruments in different positions, such as high up, stretched forward, out to one side, etc.
   d. Encourage clients to listen while only one type of instruments plays (such as all bells play or all drums play).

Individuals with profound mental retardation are going to need a great deal of physical assistance to complete the above skills. Nevertheless, this type of activity provides auditory and cognitive stimulation, and can improve gross and fine motor skills.

4. At least three times during this activity the music should be turned off and the group members encouraged to trade instruments.
5. If possible, encourage peer and/or staff interaction by cooperative instrument play:
   a. Rhythm sticks (caregiver could hold one stick and tap it against the client's stick or try to encourage two clients to tap sticks together)
   b. Drums (caregiver could strike a mallet on a drum held by a client, or vice versa. Two clients could also tap the same drum)
   c. Xylophone (same as drums)

Reminders:
1. Always encourage clients to look at and/or listen to one another.
2. Encourage choices whenever possible!
3. Make sure the music is loud enough but not blasting.
4. If an individual refuses (or is unable) to play an instrument, do not give up! Try interacting by having clients hold hands with each other and the caregivers, and move to the music in any way possible.

Music and Tactile Defensiveness

Purpose:
- Decrease/eliminate tactile defensiveness
- Stimulate interest in a shared activity
- Stimulate interest in social interaction

Materials:
- Tape/CD player and preferred music (either stimulative or sedative)

Preferred Setting:
Although this activity needs to be one-on-one with the client, a group setting in a circle is ideal. You can work with one person, while the other group members are playing instruments or doing another activity where music is already playing. The group setting is ideal because the client has the opportunity to see his/her peers at all times. If the client is visually impaired or blind, this activity also works well.

Procedure:
This is an easy activity, but it requires patience and time. (It will not be successful in a short period of time.) Sit in front of the client and follow this procedure each time you do this activity:

1. Choose music the client prefers, if possible. Allow the client to listen to the music for a minute or two while you occasionally make your presence known either by talking or by touching the client's leg, trunk, etc. (A part of the body where touch is known to be more readily tolerated by that person.)
2. Next, take one of the client's hands with a firm grip. If the client starts to pull away, immediately apply deep pressure to the palm. If the client continues to pull away, allow him/her to do so, but keep repeating this procedure. You will have to use your good judgment here.
3. If (or when!) the client begins to relax, loosen your grip a little bit and perhaps move the client's arm back and forth gently to the beat of the music.
4. Repeat this procedure with the other hand, if possible. Both hands together, moving and dancing, is your goal, but have patience!

Reminders:
If the client will not allow hand-holding at all, try starting with a backrub (deep pressure) or just touching the client's head, trunk, or legs.

Vibration

Purpose:
- To increase awareness of body parts
- To provide tactile stimulation
- To promote relaxation
- To encourage manipulation of objects with hands

Materials:
- Handheld vibrators
- Vibrating snakes/tubes (see Part 3 for resources)
- Vibrating pillows

Preferred Setting:
This activity can occur anywhere, but it is preferable for the individuals to be in a position that allows maximal access to body parts and skin.

Procedure:
1. Ensure that the client is positioned comfortably, then explain the activity.
2. If the person is positioned on his/her back, apply vibration to the following areas in this order:
   - Upper Chest
   - Arms
   - Legs
   - Cheeks
3. If the person is positioned on his/her stomach, apply vibration to the following areas in this order:
   - Back
   - Arms
   - Legs
   - Cheeks (if accessible)
5. The client should also be encouraged to:
   - *a.* apply the vibrator to his/her own body parts as independently as possible;
   - *b.* manipulate the vibrating objects with his/her hands.

Reminders:
1. Vibration is a powerful stimulus! Watch for signs of over-stimulation (e.g., agitation, withdrawal).
2. Avoid vibration over bones near the surface of the skin (i.e., wrist, hands, feet, ankles) or over body cavities (i.e., eyes, mouth, abdomen).

Texture Rub

Purpose:
- To increase awareness of body parts
- To provide tactile stimulation
- To increase manipulation with hands
- To encourage tactile discrimination (discriminate between objects by the way they feel)

Materials:
- Texture rub kit: a collection of swatches of fabric with distinct and different textures (velvet, sandpaper, lambs wool, flannel, burlap, terry cloth, chenille, cotton, etc.)

Preferred Setting:
This activity can occur anywhere, but it is preferable for the individual to be in a position that allows maximal access to exposed skin (arms, hands, legs, neck, face).

Procedure:
1. Ensure that the individual is positioned comfortably.
2. Explain the activity to the individual.
3. Rub the person's skin with the first fabric swatch using slow movements. Be gentle, especially with rougher fabrics.
4. While rubbing, talk to the individual about the fabric. Describe how it should feel, ask whether the person likes the way it feels, talk about the articles of clothing or items that might be made from this fabric, etc.
5. After rubbing all available areas of skin with the first fabric, repeat steps two through four with the second contrasting fabric.
6. After the completion of the second fabric swatch, place both pieces of fabric near the person's hands and encourage the feeling/manipulation of these swatches with one or both hands. If the individual is unable to reach for these swatches, then place them directly in his/her hands.

Reminders:
1. Watch for signs of tactile defensiveness (pulling away, crying, agitation). If this persists, either stop the activity or try to find a fabric that is not offensive.
2. Encourage independence whenever possible. At some point during this activity see if the individual will make an attempt to rub the fabric on his/her arms or hands.

Brushing

Purpose:
- To provide tactile sensory stimulation
- To increase awareness of body parts
- To increase tolerance of appropriate social touch

Materials:
- A variety of soft bristle brushes (e.g., baby hair brush, paint brush, soft clothing brush, etc.)

Preferred Setting:
This activity can be implemented in any setting but requires maximal access to exposed skin on various body parts.

Procedure:
1. Place the individual in a comfortable position.
2. Brush any exposed skin on the person's body with a brush, using slow movements. Be sure to use only downward strokes (do not brush against the direction that the hair grows!)
3. While brushing, talk to the individual about the body part being brushed or about the type of brush being used.
4. Encourage the individual to brush the identified body parts by himself/herself.

Reminders:
1. Brushing is a strong stimulus! Watch for signs of over-stimulation (i.e. agitation or withdrawal), especially if you brush against the direction of the body hair.
2. Be very attentive to the choice of brushes. Inappropriate brushes (such as ones with hard bristles) could cause skin damage.
3. If you are working with a client who has difficulty relaxing, try adding sedative type music in the background to create a calmer atmosphere.

Deep Massage

Purpose:
- To increase awareness of body parts
- To increase tolerance of social touch

Materials:
None needed

Preferred Setting:
This activity can occur anywhere, but the individual should be positioned to allow maximal access to the body parts indicated in the procedure section.

Procedure:

1. Ensure that the individual is positioned comfortably and explain the activity.
2. Apply firm, deep pressure slowly with open hands in the following sequence—
   If the client is positioned on his/her back:
   > Shoulders
   > Upper Chest
   > Arms
   > Hands
   > Hips
   > Legs
   > Feet

   If the client is positioned on his/her stomach or seated:
   > Shoulders
   > Back
   > Arms
   > Hands
   > Hips
   > Legs
   > Feet

3. Follow this sequence until the person has received at least one minute of deep massage/relaxation on each body area. This may be repeated.

Reminders:

1. During this scenario, use music that is sedative in nature (quiet, soothing). This may initially produce a relaxed state and increase the effect of the deep massage.
2. Watch for signs of tactile defensiveness (e.g., pulling away, crying, agitation). If this persists, stop the activity.
3. Deep massage is not relaxing unless it is done slowly!
4. If you are working in a group, you could encourage other individuals to watch what you are doing, or perhaps give them something to manipulate while they are listening to sedative music, such as the scarves used with the Scenario titled "Movement with Ribbon Sticks/Scarves" in the Gross Motor section.

Water Exploration

Purpose:
- To provide exposure to a variety of visual and tactile sensory stimulation
- To provide exposure to variations in temperature
- To improve functional motion of arms and hands
- To increase ability to follow simple directions
- To encourage eye-hand coordination

Materials:
- Basins
- Sponges of various sizes, shapes and textures
- Small manipulatives and objects (both those that float and sink)
- Liquid soap (to provide bubbles)
- Ice (for exploring temperature variations)
- Small containers that hold water

Preferred Setting:
Tabletop or at a sink

Procedure:
1. Encourage the clients to participate in as much of the activity preparation as possible (e.g., holding the basin, turning on the water). Physical assistance should be offered only when necessary.
2. Encourage the clients to place the sponges, manipulatives, and/or soap in the water.
3. Provide the opportunity for the clients to explore the water independently. You may need to demonstrate or provide physical assistance if there is initial difficulty.
4. Encourage each individual to use his/her hands to explore the water in any of the following ways:
   a. Squeeze water out of the sponges.
   b. Pour water from one container to another.
   c. Push objects under the water or across the surface of the water.
   d. Move hands to create soap bubbles.

Reminders:
1. If a client has an open wound, he/she should not participate in this activity.
2. Be very cautious of water temperature, especially if you are incorporating ice cubes into the activity.
3. Be creative and use other items in the water, if you feel they might be more motivating, but remember that children's water toys are not age-appropriate for adults.

Sponges

Purpose:
- To increase exposure to a variety of visual and tactile sensory stimuli.
- To increase grip strength in hands
- To improve gross motor motions of upper extremities
- To reinforce elementary self care or homemaking tasks

Materials:
- Portable basins or double-basin sink
- A variety of different colored, texture, and size sponges (loofah, sea sponge, kitchen sponge, etc.)
- Towels

Preferred Setting:
Set up portable basins at a table of appropriate height. If you are utilizing sink, make sure there is adequate open space underneath for clients using wheelchairs.

If you are emphasizing the self-care piece of the activity, you may want to consider structuring the group in the normal setting for bathing.

Procedure:
1. Position the materials, or client, for the desired effect (*close* for those with physical limitations or *away* to encourage active movement of arms through maximal range).

2. Fill one basin with warm water. Keep the other dry. This is the time to use your creativity to change the water into a sensory material. You could do one of the following:
   a. Add bubblebath to water for additional tactile, visual and olfactory (smell) input.
   b. Add food coloring for additional visual stimulus.
   c. Add baby oil or lotion to condition the skin.
   d. Heat water, or add ice cubes, to change the temperature of the water.
   Combine any of the above or try your own ideas.
3. Place a variety of sponges of different sizes, textures or colors in the wet basin. Clients should be encouraged to explore the water and sponges. As the group facilitator, encourage clients to feel the different textured sponges. Provide appropriate assistance to people with physical limitations. Try some of the following variations:
   a. Clients could drain water into the "dry" basin by squeezing water out of the sponge.
   b. To emphasize self-care, a client could do mock-bathing by wiping face, arms, or any exposed skin with the sponge. Clients can then use the towel to wipe away applied water.
   c. To encourage homemaking, clients could wipe the tabletop or sink surface, walls, or other surfaces with the sponge.

Reminders:
1. If a client has an open wound, he/she should not participate in this activity.
2. If you are using heated or chilled water, be sure to test the temperature on your skin first.
3. Encourage socialization at all times by encouraging clients to look at each other.
4. Be aware that some individuals may be allergic to food coloring.

Walking

Purpose:
- To increase awareness of the outdoors
- To provide a variety of visual, tactile and olfactory sensory stimuli
- To encourage socialization
- To increase ambulation or wheelchair propulsion skills
- To increase exposure to traffic safety rules

Materials:
None needed. This activity encompasses anything that is outdoors in the environment

Procedure:
The significance of this scenario is the quality of social interaction between you and the individual, rather than the physical activity it involves. You might want to incorporate any of the following ideas into the activity to increase the social component:

   a. Talk to the individual about sights, sounds and weather.
   b. Physically point out interesting sights during the walk.
   c. If the client is ambulatory, ask the individual to imitate you as you adhere to simple street safety signs.
   d. Place your arm around the individual, or walk arm-in-arm during the walk.
   e. Collect items for the Nature Box Scenario.

Reminders:
1. Stress awareness of the outside environment by discussing the appropriateness of clothes while you prepare for the walk.
2. Remember the age of the people with whom you are walking. If you hold hands with an individual it can appear as if you are walking with a child. Consider how you would walk with an older parent, but also consider the comfort and safety of the client.
3. If you find yourself at a loss for environmental topics, talk about your day, your last vacation, the client's evening activity, a good movie, etc. The important factor, as stated above, is the quality of the interaction. Eventually, as you continue to walk, you will find new aspects of the environment to discuss.

CHAPTER 7

Gross Motor

1. Shoulder Arc

2. Movement With Ribbon Sticks and Scarves

3. "Play the Xylophone"

4. Hokey Pokey

5. Dance/Movement With Chinese Jumprope

6. Therapy Balls

7. Beanbag "Basketball"

8. Obstacle Course

Shoulder Arc

Purpose:
- To increase/maintain range of motion of shoulders
- To improve gross motor motions of arms
- To encourage development of fine motor skills
- To encourage eye-hand coordination

Materials:
Shoulder Arc (See Part 3 for resources)

Preferred Setting:
The Shoulder Arc should be placed on a table of appropriate height depending on whether the client is sitting or standing

Procedure:
1. Position the individual in front of the Shoulder Arc, either standing or sitting.
2. Encourge the individual to reach and grasp one colored piece on the Arc.
3. Encourage the individual to move the colored piece to the other side of the arc with as much independent movement as possible. (Use physical assistance only if absolutely necessary.)
4. Continue to encourage the individual to move all the colored pieces from one side of the Arc to the other.
5. When all the pieces have been moved, start the process over, but encourage the individual to use his/her other arm to return the pieces.

Reminders:
1. Since only one person can use the Shoulder Arc at a time, ensure group involvement by encouraging clients to look at the person using the Arc. You could also encourage taking turns by having several clients move different pieces on the Arc.
2. If you choose to use background music during this activity, choose music that will encourage fluid movement of arms (i.e., anything that does not have a steady, driving beat).
3. If you are not sure whether the clients can reach the height of the Arc, consult with an occupational therapist.

Movement With Ribbon Sticks and Scarves

Purpose:
- Increase available range of motion
- Increase visual tracking
- Increase awareness of peers
- Maintain grasp of an object (increase grip strength)

Materials:
- Ribbon Sticks (Easy to make! See Part 3 for instructions)
- Scarves (Best to use chiffon. These can be found at local thrift shops or yard sales.)
- Choice of recorded music: Recommended for a quiet activity: sedative-type music such as New Age or soft classical music with a slow tempo Recommended for a lively activity: stimulative-type music such as 1950s rock 'n' roll, Bluegrass, etc.
- Tape/CD player

Preferred Setting:
Clients should be seated in a large circle (one arm's length apart). Spacing allows the caregiver enough room to move in and out of the circle as needed to assist the clients from a variety of directions without impeding their view.

Procedure:
1. The caregiver should give each client a ribbon stick or scarf (or encourage them to choose one, if possible).
2. The caregiver should choose music according to need and have a client assist with turning it on. (Switches can be used very effectively here!)
3. The caregiver should encourage the following types of movement:
   a. Lift the ribbon/scarf high up in the air
   b. Move the ribbon/scarf from side to side
   c. Move the ribbon/scarf rapidly
   d. Move the ribbon/scarf slowly
   e. Hold and move the ribbon/scarf with two hands together
   f. Hold and move the ribbon/scarf with each hand alone
   g. Touch toes with the ribbon/scarf

Be creative here! Try to encourage any kind of independent movement. Perhaps visual tracking will be the major goal for some group members. If possible, try to encourage clients to interact with each other by having two people hold the opposite end of the same scarf and manipulate it together.

Reminders:
1. Always encourage movement through available range. Consult with the Occupational and/or physical therapist to determine abilities, limitations, and special needs. (Often we tend to limit clients more than is necessary for fear we will hurt them.)
2. The type of music you choose will affect the behavior of the clients. Use the music to suit your needs; consider such factors as the energy level you wish to create and the personal preferences of the clients. (Or perhaps the caregivers, if that will ensure more participation!)
3. To foster group involvement, clients should be encouraged to look at each other as much as possible.
4. If clients are unable to grasp the scarf, try tying it around their hand, arm or finger. You can also secure a piece of elastic to one end as a loop. Adaptive devices can be created or purchased for the ribbon sticks (see Part 3).

"Play the Xylophone"

Purpose:
- Increase gross motor skills
- Maintain grasp of an object (grip strength)
- Increase eye-hand coordination
- Develop a leisure skill

Materials: (See Part 3 for resources)
- Xylophone (any size)
- Mallet (with built-up handle or adaptive strap if needed)

Preferred Setting:
If you are using a large xylophone, the client should be seated in front of a low table so that the top of the xylophone is approximately at waist level. If you are using a small xylophone, a regular table or wheelchair tray can be used. If this is a group activity, seat clients so that two of them can reach the xylophone, preferably facing each other.

Procedure:
1. Place the mallet in the client's hand and encourage him/her to play independently. Use physical assistance only as needed.
2. If physical assistance is required, try to play a well-known song. (The letter names are on the bars of the xylophone, and you can easily learn the two simple songs in the next column.)

AMAZING GRACE

A - maz ing Grace
C F   AF   A

How sweet the sound
G   F   D C

That saved a wretch like me
C F   AF A   G C

I once was lost
A C A C A F

But now - I'm found
C   D   FD C

Was blind - but now I see
C   F   AF A G C

ROW ROW ROW YOUR BOAT

Row row row your boat
C   C   C D   E

Gent - ly down - the stream
E   D   E   F   G

Mer-ri-ly
C C

Mer-ri-ly
G G

Mer-ri-ly
E EE

Mer-ri-ly
C CC

Life is but a dream
G F E D C

3. Encourage independence (fade the physical prompts). If necessary, position the xylophone a different way to make it easier for the client to reach and play.

Reminders:
You can use background music if you wish (if not playing a structured song). You will know best what your clients might enjoy or what might increase participation. Play it loud enough to hear, but do not drown out the xylophone sounds.

Hokey Pokey

Purpose:
- Increase gross motor skills (range of motion)
- Develop/increase skills in following simple directions
- Increase awareness of peers
- Develop/increase imitation skills
- Increase awareness of body parts

Materials:
- Tape/CD player
- Tape of Hokey Pokey or live music (see Part 3 for resources)

Preferred Setting:
Large circle with enough room for caregivers to stand, sit beside, or move freely in and around the clients in the circle.

Procedure:
1. Begin by turning on the tape of the Hokey Pokey (you can also sing this and make up any movements suitable for the clients). You do not need instruments—just your voice is enough. If you choose to sing, do so very slowly.
2. Each caregiver should interact with one client for the entire song and then move on to another client and do the same.
3. Physically assist clients if they are unable to do the requested movements. This activity should flow like a dance activity.
4. For each verse of the song, there is a command: "put your right foot in, put your right foot out" and then a Hokey Pokey line; "Do the Hokey Pokey and turn yourself around." During the Hokey Pokey part of the music you should either continue the commanded movement or just dance with the client. (Move his/her body as much as possible.)
5. For the command "Put your whole self in," if the client uses a wheelchair you should move it forward and back or around. If the client does not use a wheelchair and has limited mobility, move his/her body as much as possible.

Reminders:
Be creative. Create different movements to keep the activity interesting. If possible, ask the clients to create movements (or use movements they are already doing.) You can also include props, such as musical instruments ("Put the bell in"…)

Dance/ Movement With Chinese Jumprope

Purpose:
• Increase gross motor movement
• Increase participation in a group activity
• Facilitate grasping skills
• Maintain grip strength

Materials:
• Chinese Jumprope, Co-Oper Band™ (see Part 3 for resources), or any alternative to a large stretchy loop (see Part 3 for ideas)
• CD/tape player, utilizing lively music

Preferred Setting:
Clients should be seated in a circle, approximately the same size as the stretch band. Caregivers should be seated next to those individuals who might need assistance.

Procedure:
1. Turn on lively music.
2. Encourage each client to grasp the stretch band with both hands.
3. Encourage the group to do the following:
   a. Pull the stretch band back and forth, toward and away from their bodies.
   b. Raise the stretch band up and bring it down again.
   c. Slide the stretch band through their hands so it moves around the circle.
   d. Move the stretch band forward and around in a circular motion.
   e. Try any other movement you can invent.

Reminders:
1. This activity is primarily for gross motor movement. Repeat the above movements many times—it is good exercise.
2. Always encourage people to look at each other and to be aware of who is seated next to whom. Use every opportunity to increase peer awareness.

Therapy Balls

GROSS MOTOR

Purpose:
- To improve functional movements of arms and legs
- To increase visual tracking
- To increase socialization with caregivers and peers

Materials:
- Large therapy ball, standing taller than knee height (see Part 3 for resources)

Preferred Setting:
Clients should be seated in a large circle in a room, or outside with a lot of space. If possible, caregivers should be seated within the circle, next to the clients.

Procedure:
1. After everyone is seated in a large circle, you should stand in the center of the circle to control the motion of the ball.
2. Provide an explanation of the activity (e.g., "John, I'm going to roll the ball to you.")
3. Slowly roll the ball to the client, and verbally encourage the client to catch the ball.
4. Ask the client to roll the ball back to the center of the circle or to another member of the group. Suggest different ways to move the ball, such as kicking it or pushing it. If the individual is having difficulty, offer assistance as needed.
5. Encourage all the members of the group to watch the movement of the ball.

Reminders:
Use hand-over-hand assistance only when necessary. Independent movement of any kind should be encouraged.

Beanbag "Basketball"

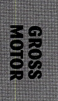

Purpose:
- Increase gross motor movement
- Increase visual tracking
- Facilitate grasp and release skill
- Increase awareness of peers
- Increase participation in group activity

Materials:
- Variety of beanbags (preferably in different colors)
- Large tambourine with a head (like a drum)

Preferred Setting:
Clients should be seated facing each other in two lines, close enough for beanbag toss. It is preferable to have two caregivers to facilitate steps one to four.

Procedure:
1. Starting with one pair of clients each facing each other, give one client the tambourine to hold (upside down, to catch the beanbag). If the client is unable to hold the tambourine, physically assist as needed.
2. Give the client opposite several beanbags to throw, demonstrating that they should be aimed at the tambourine.
3. For each bean bag that correctly goes into the tambourine, give the tambourine an extra "shake" to reinforce the musical sound of the instrument. (You could also assist the client in shaking the tambourine to make this musical sound.)
4. If you have clients that can do this, increase the distance required to throw the beanbag to make it more challenging.

Reminders:
1. If you have only one caregiver, he/she should hold the tambourine and encourage each client to throw (or place) the beanbag in the tambourine.
2. Always reinforce the correct throw of the beanbag with lots of tambourine shakes.
3. Encourage clients to look at each other as they do this activity.
4. Do not use any background music. This activity is noisy and any other sound will be distracting.

Obstacle Course

Purpose:
- To improve functional movements of head, trunk, arms and/or legs
- To provide exposure to spatial directives (up/down, on/off, right/left, etc.)
- To encourage the following of simple directions
- To increase awareness of body parts

Materials:
- Traffic cones, ropes, poles, chairs, tables, tunnels (or the addition of balls, wedges or anything that might make an obstacle course more interesting)

Preferred Setting:
Large room with a lot of empty floor space

Procedure:
1. Set up the room to create an interesting course for clients to move through. Individuals should have the opportunity to move under, over, around and through various objects. Encourage individuals to participate in this set up as much as possible.
2. Encourage individuals to move through the obstacle course with as much independence as possible (whether or not the person uses a wheelchair).
3. Expand the obstacle course to include more activities. For example, there could be stations added to the course where individuals would be encouraged to:
   a. throw, roll or kick a ball over, under, through and/or into an obstacle;
   b. place a hoop or ring onto a cone;
   c. stack cardboard boxes;
   d. place a designated body part on an obstacle;
   e. push the obstacle a designated distance across the floor or a table.

Reminders:
1. If you add background music to this activity, choose music that will encourage movement. You could add a tape player at one station and encourage clients to change the music by using a switch.
2. Be creative! This activity has a lot of room for expansion.

CHAPTER 8

Fine Motor

1. Therapeutic Putty

2. Sand Box

3. Manipulation Box

4. Egg Shaker Chant

5. Magnets

6. Peg-Board

7. Bright Builders

8. Containers

9. Lock Board

10. Collages

11. Stamp Collection

12. Flower Arranging

13. Pre-writing

Therapeutic Putty

Purpose:
- To improve hand strength
- To improve functional movements of hands/fingers
- To provide tactile stimulation

Materials:
- Commercially available therapeutic putty (see Part 3 for resources— recipe for making therapeutic putty at home is also included)

Preferred Setting:
Tabletop

Procedure:
1. Distribute a generous portion of putty to each client in the group.
2. Encourage the clients to do any of the following actions with the putty:
   a. Squeeze it in hand
   b. Flatten with open hand
   c. Pound it with fist
   d. Poke fingers into it or through it
   e. Pinch/rip small pieces off the large piece
   f. Mold it into a specific shape
3. Encourage the clients to do the above tasks as independently as possible. If someone has difficulty, provide the appropriate amount of assistance. Encourage creativity! If the client successfully manipulates the putty with a new appropriate action, reinforce this new action.
4. Talk to the clients about the putty— color, texture, shape, etc. Encourage clients to look at each other's projects.

Reminders:
If you choose to preserve the putty as artwork at some point, encourage the clients to continue to look at their artwork periodically. You could also encourage them to feel the difference between the hardened putty and the pliable putty.

Sandbox

Purpose:
- To improve functional movements of hands/fingers
- To provide tactile and/or visual stimulation
- To reinforce the concept of object permanence
- To provide exposure to the use of hand tools
- To reinforce simple spatial concepts (under, in, out, etc.)

Materials:
- Containers of various sizes depending upon the range of activities you wish to encourage (e.g., a sand bucket for exploration with fingers or a large box, if you wish to include the use of tools to fill other smaller containers with sand)
- Sand (or you can substitute rice, dry beans, styrofoam packing pellets, etc.) Sand can be purchased in large bags from a plant nursery/landscaping store
- Objects to place in the sand, that are in various shapes, sizes and colors
- Spoons, handheld shovels or rakes (optional for this activity)

Preferred Setting:
Tabletop

Procedure:
1. Place all of the materials for this activity on the table. Begin by placing the sand, (rice, beans, et al.) in various containers.
2. Encourage each client to manipulate the materials as follows:
   a. move fingers through the various textured materials in the containers (describe each item to the clients as they do this);
   b. remove objects placed (or hidden) in the sand;
   c. pour sand from one container to another or through a strainer into a container;
   d. spoon or shovel sand from one container to another using some containers that create challenges due to size and shape;
   e. rake sand on a flat or shallow surface (for visual and tactile stimulation).
3. Encourage group interaction as follows:
   a. Group clients in pairs and encourage one to hold the container and one to spoon or shovel.
   b. Group clients in pairs and have them move their fingers through the same large box. If their hands touch, point out who they are touching.
4. Once the task is mastered, this can become a more functional activity, e.g., pouring cereal, rice or other foods from boxes into storage containers for the kitchen.

Reminders:
To ensure that this activity is age-appropriate, do not use children's sand shovels, buckets, etc. Be creative! You can use many interesting household items such as collanders, sifters and pitchers.

Note: once the household items are taken outside, they must be cleaned and disenfected throughly before they are used with food preparation again.

Manipulation Box

Purpose:
- To encourage manipulation of objects with one or both hands
- To improve fine motor grasp of small objects
- To increase eye-hand coordination
- To increase exposure to a variety of tactile stimuli

Materials:
- Manipulation Box (consisting of a variety of small objects). The objects should encourage manipulation by one hand alone or by both hands at the same time. The kit should include these objects:

  Unilateral Use(with one hand): checkers, pencil, marbles, tennis ball, feather.

  Bilateral Use (with two hands): dowel (large stick), large ball, book/magazine, large drum, rainstick (see Part 3 for resources)

Preferred Setting:
Tabletop

Procedure:
1. Cue the client to select an item and remove it from the box. Position the box so the client has to reach through maximal range purposefully. Utilize the least amount of physical assistance necessary.
2. Give clients enough time to explore the selected item independently.
3. Talk to each client about the object they are holding (e.g., "I see you have a pencil. It's a yellow pencil. Show me what you can do with the pencil.")
4. Be alert for signs of waning attention from the client (e.g., a decrease in visual attention to the object or a decrease in movement of the hands). Periodically encourage clients to exchange items with other group members.
5. Encourage manipulation of small objects with both hands.
6. Encourage selection of larger objects that would require bilateral manipulation (both hands at the same time).
7. If using a kit that contains self-care items, have the client talk about or imitate their use.

Reminders:
1. Try to encourage functional manipulation (not self-stimulatory behaviors such as flapping, twirling, etc.)
2. Be creative! Find items for your kits that are different from the objects individuals use on a daily basis. This is a great opportunity for new experiences.
3. Encourage socialization through the exchange of objects by asking each person to look at each other, etc.

Egg Shaker Chant

Purpose:
- Increase fine motor skills
- Increase gross motor skills
- Participate in a group activity
- Maintain grip strength

Materials:
- Egg shakers (see Part 3 for resources)

Preferred Setting:
Clients should be seated in a circle facing each other. There should be enough room for caregivers to move in and out of the circle as needed, or to sit next to people.

Procedure:

1. Demonstrate/model the sound of the egg shaker. This is a good opportunity to have the client locate the sound source and then visually track it.
2. Give the client the opportunity to reach out for the egg shaker and grasp it.
3. If the client does not reach for the egg shaker, place it in his/her hand.
4. Assist the client in shaking the egg shaker while providing the stimulus of a simple chant. You can make up a chant, or use one of these chants below. The important part is to keep a steady beat going while you speak the words.

Chant 1
Music, music all around,
Shake the egg and hear the sound
Shake it high, shake it low
Shake the egg from head to toe

Chant 2
Shake it up, Shake it up
Shake it and play
You're doing great
Makin' music today

Reminders:

1. While clients are shaking the eggs, take the opportunity to move their arms up and down, from side to side, etc. Consult the occupational therapist or physical therapist to ensure that maximum arm range is not exceeded.
2. If you are not comfortable chanting, use recorded music. It must have a good steady beat, and it should not be played louder than the sounds of the egg shakers.

FINE MOTOR

Magnets

FINE MOTOR

Purpose:
- To improve functional movement of hands/fingers
- To improve eye-hand coordination
- To provide tactile and visual stimulation
- To reinforce basic spatial concepts

Materials:
- Magnets of various sizes, shapes, and colors that can be purchased commercially. You can also purchase magnets that come in particular sets (such as flowers, animals, etc.), and these can be grouped together to emphasize classification skills
- Magnet Board or flat metal surface, such as a refrigerator or cabinet door, or cookie sheet
- Plastic container to store magnets

Preferred Setting:
Close proximity to a metal surface. If you have a group of people, ensure that everyone can see others engaged in the activity.

Procedure:
1. Open the plastic box containing the magnets and encourage each client in your group to choose and remove several magnets. Assist the clients in placing these magnets in front of themselves on the table, picture side up.
2. Place the magnet board in front of each client and encourage them to do any of the following:
   a. Attach the magnet to the board.
   b. Slide the magnet along the edge of the board, up and down, or from side to side (you can also draw a path for them to follow).
   c. Pull the magnet off the board.
3. As a variation to this activity, try any of the following:
   a. Place the magnet board at a greater distance away from the client to encourage reaching and stretching.
   b. Encourage clients to group types of magnets together on the board (such as colors, foods, animals, sports items, flowers, etc.).
   c. Encourage clients to utilize magnets functionally in their environment by having them use a magnet to hang a photo or artwork on the refrigerator.
   d. Illustrate the difference between metallic and nonmetallic surfaces by asking clients to place the magnets on different surfaces.
   e. Encourage taking turns and sharing within the group through passing magnets to each other, having one client hold the magnetic surface for another, etc.

Reminders:
1. Consult the occupational therapist or physical therapist if stretching or reaching is encouraged, so maximum aim range is not exceeded.
2. Always encourage clients to look at each other during this activity and to socialize as much as possible.

Peg-Board

Purpose:
- To increase fine motor skills
- To improve eye-hand coordination
- To encourage problem-solving skills
- To encourage socialization with peers

Materials:
- Peg-Board (These can be purchased from specialized catalogs or can be handmade. See Part 3 for resources and ideas.)

Preferred Setting:
Tabletop

Procedure:
1. Place the peg-board and the container of pegs directly in front of the client.
2. Demonstrate the correct way to place the pegs into the board. If there are pegs of various sizes or shapes, encourage the client to manipulate each one.
3. Encourage the client to place the pegs in the matching holes of the peg-board. Provide assistance only if necessary.
4. If you would like to encourage peer interaction, place a peg-board between two individuals and encourage them to take turns placing the pegs into the holes.
5. If you would like to encourage learning in other areas, try these variations:
   a. Use colored pegs and encourage clients to match the the colored peg to the same colored hole.
   b. Circle some of the holes with a Magic Marker and encourage clients to place pegs only into the marked holes.
   c. Increase the difficulty of the task by creating or purchasing a peg-board with smaller pegs and holes.

Reminders:
The main purpose of this activity is to develop and/or increase fine motor skills. If the client is not even able to grasp the peg, you will have to begin by working with just this small part of the task.

Bright Builders

Purpose:
- To increase functional motions of arms and hands
- To increase awareness of spatial concepts (e.g., up/down, right/left, top/bottom, front/back, etc.)
- To increase elementary motor planning (construction) abilities
- To increase exposure to a variety of tactile and visual sensory materials
- To encourage bilateral (utilizing two/both) use of hands

Materials:
- Commercially available Bright Builders (see Part 3 for resources) or other connecting blocks.

Preferred Setting:
Tabletop

Procedure:
1. Encourge clients to remove one block at a time from the box. If the client has difficulty, offer assistance only as needed.
2. Ensure that all the blocks are distributed among the group members.
3. Encourage clients to watch you as you demonstrate how to connect the blocks together.
4. Encourage clients to begin to build with the blocks. Individuals can build their own structures or can take turns adding to a group structure. Always encourage as much independence as possible and offer assistance only if necessary.
5. After all blocks are used and the structure is complete, encourage clients to watch as you demonstrate how to pull the blocks apart.
6. Encourage clients to begin to take apart the structure. Again, encourage as much independence as possible and give assistance only when necessary.

Reminders:
If you are unable to find or purchase Bright Builders, you can substitute other commercially produced connecting blocks. Age appropriate items are available, especially in stores that sell leisure items for adults.

Containers

Purpose:
- To improve ability to use hands/fingers functionally to open various types of containers
- To improve bilateral use of arms
- To improve eye-hand coordination
- To reinforce simple spatial/directional concepts, e.g. on/off, in/out, etc.

Materials:
- Collection of containers with various types of lids (twist off, pull off, flip top) and in various shapes and sizes. Containers should be organized into a "kit" to provide individuals with multiple opportunities to manipulate containers functionally during a set time period.
- Sensory stimulation objects that can be placed in each container (e.g., swatches of fabric, rice, beans, aromatic objects, small objects to manipulate, etc.)

Preferred Setting:
Tabletop

Procedure:
1. Encourage the client to manipulate each container as independently as possible.
2. Provide hand-over-hand assistance to those individuals with physical challenges or simplify the task so the person can be successful (e.g., loosen a screw-off lid, pry up a corner of a plastic pull-off lid).
3. Talk to the client about the type of container with which they are working. Discuss the action needed to open the container or what type of items the container would normally hold.
4. Once the container is open, encourage the client to place various types of objects into it with their hands or appropriate tools (such as a spoon).
5. Encourage the client to replace the lid on the container. This is an important part of the task, but it is developmentally more difficult. Again, hand-over-hand assistance or simplification of the task can be used to encourage independence.
6. It would be beneficial to follow up this activity with practical hands-on manipulation of the same types of containers in their normal environment (e.g., kitchen containers).

Reminders:
1. Caution should be used when using glass containers.
2. Remember that it is more beneficial for a client to complete a small piece of the task successfully than to keep struggling with the entire procedure.
3. Encourage clients to observe each other as one person completes the task.
4. This scenario can be combined with the scenarios titled Sandbox, (Fine Motor 2) and/or Manipulation Box (Fine Motor 3).

Lock Board

Purpose:
- To practice manipulation of various types of locks and/or environmental control devices (faucets, light switches, etc.)
- To improve functional movements of hands/fingers
- To improve eye-hand coordination

Materials:
- Commercially available or handmade lock board (see Part 3 for resources/ideas)

Preferred Setting:
Tabletop or within close proximity to a wall-mounted lock board

Procedure:
1. Encourage the client to manipulate (open/close, turn on/off, move) each object on the lock board as independently as possible.
2. Provide assistance to those individuals with physical challenges or simplify each task, so the person can be successful (e.g., instead of unlocking the padlock and removing it from the board, you may just want to have the client turn the key or lift the open lock off the board).
3. Talk to the client about the object with which they are working. Explain it's purpose or where in the environment the object can be found. Encourage other clients in your group to observe the task and the objects.
4. It would be beneficial to follow up this activity with practical hands-on manipulation of the same locks, faucets, etc. in their normal environment.

Reminders:
1. If you are creating your own board, you should use the same or similar objects to those found in the client's home or workplace. This board can contain many different items.
2. Remember that it is more beneficial for a client to complete a small piece of the task successfully than to keep struggling with the entire procedure.

Collages

Purpose:
- To increase fine motor skills
- To increase eye-hand coordination
- To encourage peer interaction and sharing
- To increase skills in object identification

Materials:
- Poster/construction paper
- Magazines
- Paste or glue (glue sticks would be easier to use)
- Scissors (see Part 3 for resources for adapted scissors)

Preferred Setting:
Tabletop

Procedure:
1. Place all the materials on the table and explain the activity to the clients (show the magazine pictures and explain that they will be cut out and glued to the paper).
2. Encourage each client to choose a magazine and begin looking through it for pictures. You can then move from client to client, helping each one to find one picture to be cut out. If the client is able to rip out the page, encourage him/her to do so, then assist with the cutting as needed. There are several approaches you can take with regard to the choice of pictures:
   a. Encourage clients to choose any picture in the magazine.
   b. Encourage clients to choose pictures in a specific category, such as flowers, people, food, etc.
   c. As another alternative, you can also create collages from items that have particular textures, such as cotton balls, velvet, sandpaper, etc.
3. As you work with the group, remember to talk about the activity, particularly if there is a topic that relates to the magazine pictures. When the collages are completed, have each person show their artwork to the group.
4. If possible, display the collages around the room and remind clients to look at them daily.

Reminders:
If you choose to use background music, select tapes/CD's that will create a calm environment. Music that is instrumental is preferable, so the words of the songs do not compete with your talking.

Stamp Collection

Purpose:
- To improve functional movement of hands/fingers
- To improve eye-hand coordination
- To provide visual, tactile and/or olfactory (smell) stimulation
- To provide an age-appropriate leisure experience
- To reinforce simple spatial concepts

Materials:
- Stamp album (available commercially or can be handmade)
- Stamps of various sizes, shapes, and visual appearances. (Fragrance can be added for increase sensory stimulation. Stickers can be used in place of stamps, as long as they are deemed age-appropriate. These can be purchased at office supplies stores or stationery stores with pictures/designs, or you can draw designs on solid color self-adhesive labels.)
- Sponges that can be utilized to wet the stamps, if the client is unable to lick them. Self-adhesive stamps are available commercially.

Preferred Setting:
Tabletop

Procedure:
1. Place a variety of stamps and/or stickers on the table and encourage clients to choose one/several/many for this activity. If the clients are unable to choose, place several stamps or stickers in front of them. Describe the pictures to each individual. You can group stamps/stickers together if you want to:
   a. teach individuals about the similarities of objects, colors, etc.;
   b. teach individuals the concept of size.
2. Place the stamp album in front of each individual, encouraging them to open it and turn to the first available unused page.
3. If using stamps, encourage the client to attach it to the page by licking it or by rubbing it on a wet sponge. (If you are unsure which procedure should be used, consult with an occupational therapist regarding sensitivity in the mouth area or issues regarding the use of the mouth or tongue.)
4. Once the task is mastered, this scenario can be turned into a functional activity or job, such as:
   a. Placing postal stamps on envelopes.
   b. Placing labels on items such as jars, folders, boxes, etc.
   c. Placing mailing stickers on envelopes and boxes.

Reminders:
If you are aware of a client's preference, such as bright colors or particular foods, you might want to find stamps or stickers that reinforce this preference.

Flower Arranging

Purpose:
- To improve functional movements of arms, hands and fingers
- To improve eye-hand coordination
- To provide visual, tactile and/or olfactory (smell) stimulation
- To provide an age-appropriate leisure experience
- To reinforce simple spatial concepts (in/out)

Materials:
- Real, silk or dried flowers or foliage. Be creative; use flowers of various types, sizes, colors, textures. Fragrance can be added to silk, dried or artificial flowers.
- Container or vase for the flower arrangement. You can also purchase floral foam into which flower stems can be inserted. Floral foam is available in florist shops, plant nurseries and craft supplies stores.

Preferred Setting:
Tabletop

Procedure:
1. If you choose to scent the flowers, do this prior to starting the activity.
2. Encourage clients to choose flowers for their own arrangement or the group arrangement.
3. Encourage clients to place the flowers in a vase or in floral foam to create an attractive arrangement. Ensure that everyone has the opportunity to smell the flowers as they work with them. If you are working with one person at a time, talk about what you are doing and encourage the other group members to watch.
4. When the arrangement is finished, assist the client in placing it in a preferred setting. If the individual is not capable of making this choice, assist him/her in placing the arrangement in a spot where they will see it on a daily basis.

Reminders:
1. This activity does not require much verbalization. Therefore, background music can be played to create a pleasant atmosphere. Choose music for this activity that sets the mood you want to foster.
2. Encourage the clients to look at and to smell the flower arrangements on a daily basis.

Pre-Writing

Purpose:
- To improve functional movements of hands/fingers
- To improve eye-hand coordination
- To provide visual and tactile sensory stimulus
- To reinforce basic spatial concepts
- To provide an age-appropriate leisure experience

Materials:
- Paper of various sizes, colors, textures. Paper may be bound into a book, or you can purchase a drawing/sketch book
- Age-appropriate coloring books (see Part 3 for resources)
- Age-appropriate writing or drawing utensils (e.g., pastels, Magic Markers, pen/pencils, paints and brushes)

Preferred Setting:
Tabletop

Procedure:
1. Position the paper directly in front of the client (you may want to cue the client to hold the paper/book down with the hand that is not holding the utensil).
2. Hand preference for writing is often neither set nor clear in this population. You may want to encourage grasping of the writing utensil with the one hand the individual consistently uses to hold a spoon or fork. Exploration of hand dominance by use of both hands during this activity is also acceptable.
3. Encourage normal grasp of the writing utensil. If this is difficult for the individual, you may want to consider using a writing utensil with a wider diameter. Hand-over-hand assistance to grasp the utensil is also acceptable. Use of an adaptive writing utensil may also make participation in this activity easier for the individual.
4. Be aware of the skills the client already has and encourage progression through the following developmental sequence:
   - Vertical line
   - Horizontal line
   - Crossed lines
   - Circle
   - Square
   - Triangle

Reminders:
You can draw the desired shapes yourself or have the client trace a shape design. This is sometimes beneficial in assisting the individual to draw the shape independently.

CHAPTER 9

Cognitive

1. Environmental Sounds Tape

2. Imitation

3. Body Part Identification

4. Music and Movment
   "If You're Happy and You Know It"

5. Common Object Identification

6. Find the Object

7. Making Choices

8. Memory Book

9. Puzzles

Environmental Sounds Tape

Purpose:
- To encourage environmental awareness
- To provide a variety of auditory sensory stimulation
- To improve functional motions of arms and hands
- To encourage socialization

Materials:
- Audiotapes of environmental sounds (available commercially or can be customized to include the sound of home, familiar persons, etc.)
- Tape Player
- Switch to operate tape player (optional—see Part 3 for resources)
- Pictures of items, places, people, etc. (corresponding to the sound on the tapes)

Preferred Setting:
This activity can occur anywhere but a quiet environment is preferable so there is no interference with the taped sounds.

Procedure:
1. Position the client in close proximity to the tape player.
2. Encourage the individual to place the tape in the player and turn on the tape. The client should do this with as little assistance as possible. A switch can be used, as it will create more independence.
3. While the tape is playing, encourage the client to attend to the tape by talking to him/her about the sounds being heard. You may also want to show the person pictures that correspond to the sounds being heard.

Reminders:
1. To reduce the passive nature of this activity, you can ask the client to imitate a common action/motion related to the sound on the tape (e.g., flap arms to imitate flying when a bird sound is heard).
2. If you are able to make your own tape, try to incorporate as many meaningful everyday sounds as you can, such as car horns, telephones, baby cries, dog barks, etc. Also incorporate any sounds that are particularly significant to the individuals with whom you work.

Imitation

Purpose:
- To teach a prerequisite behavior for enhanced communication
- To improve long term working memory
- To learn or enhance the use of social greetings

Materials:
None required

Preferred Setting:
This activity can occur anywhere but will work best or is more easily managed on an individual basis in an environment with minimal distraction.

Procedure:
Procedure:
1. Gain the client's attention.
2. Perform a gesture and ensure that the client is attending to your gesture. Examples of gestures are:
   a. Raising or clapping your hands
   b. Waving good-bye
   c. Using a sign (e.g., ASL)
3. With the lowest level of assistance required, encourage the client to perform the same gesture:
   a. Raise the client's hands with your hands.
   b. Assist the client with waving one hand while you wave your other hand.
   c. Manipulate the client's hands to form the sign.
4. Reinforce the client with verbal and gestural praise.
5. Repeat steps one through four.

Reminders:
1. This activity can be carried out within a group. Encourage clients to wave to each other and to attend to each other's gestures.
2. Encourage clients to imitate these or other behaviors throughout their day, if possible. Keep it simple.

Body Parts Identification

COGNITIVE

Purpose:
- To increase awareness of body parts
- To increase ability to follow directions
- To provide visual and tactile stimulus
- To reinforce concept of or orientation to self
- To improve functional movements of arms
- To encourage movement of identified body parts

Materials:
- Mirrors of various sizes (hand held, table top, or wall mounted may be appropriate depending on your goal for the activity)
- Tactile medium (shaving cream, nontoxic paint, swatches of fabric, items of clothing)

Preferred Setting:
The client needs to be in close proximity to the mirror, if a mirror is being utilized for this task. If not, a bathroom or bedroom would be the appropriate environment, if you would like to incorporate this activity into the daily self-care routine.

Procedure:
1. This activity can be composed of a variety of individual tasks that would encourage the individual to identify his/her whole self, other persons, or specific body parts. Listed below are acceptable variations on this theme:

If the mirror is used, encourage the individuals to:
- a. Point to self in the mirror
- b. Point to the other person in the mirror
- c. Point to named body parts in the mirror
- d. Perform a motion or command
- e. Point to self, another person, or named body part while watching the action in the mirror
- f. Place shaving cream, paint, or cloth on the image of himself/herself in the mirror or on the image of another person in the mirror. Then, uncover this same image by removing the paint, shaving cream, or cloth

If the mirror is not used, encourage the individual to:
- a. Point to self
- b. Touch another person
- c. Point to named body part of self or of another person
- d. Imitate a simple motion performed by another person (e.g., waving)

2. Be sure to reinforce these concepts by stating the name of the body part or by describing the action (e.g., "Mary is touching her arm").
3. Concepts such as left and right are difficult for the developmental level of this population. Their use in the discussion component of this activity, however, should not be discouraged nor excluded.
4. Be cautious of the amount of physical assistance offered to individuals during this task. It may be difficult for them visually to distinguish whose body part is whose when hand-over-hand assistance is provided.

Reminders:
If music is used in the background, ensure that it is appropriate for the mood you wish to create. For example, you can have a high energy activity by using stimulative music and encouraging people to move the designated body part to the music, or you can use sedative music and keep the activity more relaxed. Whichever music you use, your choices should be instrumental only.

Music and Movement "If You're Happy and You Know It"

Purpose:
- Increase available range of motion
- Increase skills in following simple directions
- Increase mind-body integration through sensory stimulation and motor movement
- Improve imitation skills
- Increase self-awareness through identification of main body parts (perceptual motor skills)

Materials:
- It is highly recommended to use a taped version of this song unless there are other caregivers that can interact with clients while one person plays the music. It is possible to record the song yourself. This enables you to slow it down and choose our own actions. This song can be found in many traditional song book, but it is reproduced on the next page with its original words.

Preferred Setting:
Large circle with enough room between clients for the staff to move in and out of the circle and around the group members. (The individuals can be assisted from behind and from either side, so their view is not blocked.)

Procedure:
You should interact with one client from your group for several body movements or the entire song. The song is then repeated until all clients have participated. (If you are fortunate to have a one-to-one caregiver/client ratio, all clients can participate in the song at the same time.) For the song that was created, the following actions were used:

a. "If You're Happy And You Know It, Clap Your Hands"

b. "If You're Happy And You Know It, Wave Your Arms"

c. "If You're Happy And You Know It, Tap Your Knees"

d. "If You're Happy And You Know It, Look At Me"

e. "If You're Happy And You Know It, Give A Smile"

f. "If You're Happy And You Know It, Sing With Me"

g. "If You're Happy And You Know It, Shake My Hand"

Create your own movements that would work best with your population. This song can be designed to work on specific individualized skills, or general group skills.

Reminders:
1. Always encourage movement through available range. Consult with the occupational therapist and/or physical therapist to determine abilities, limitations, and special needs. (Clients are limited by staff members more than is necessary for fear they will be hurt.)
2. Clients should be encouraged to watch each other while one member of their group is participating. (These individuals could be offered an instrument to play or verbally encouraged to do the action requested in the song.)
3. Be careful not to play the music too loud.

If You're Happy

Traditional Melody

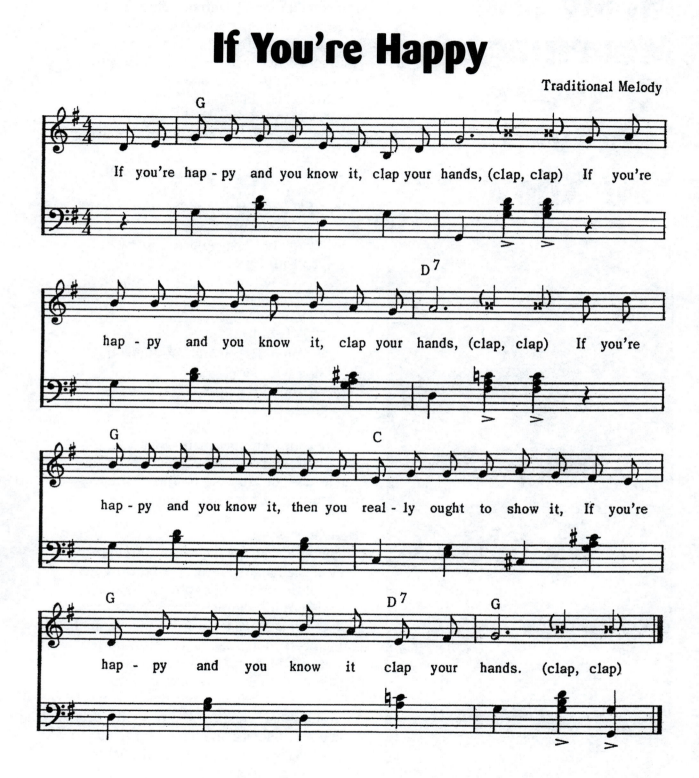

If you're hap-py and you know it, clap your hands, (clap, clap) If you're

hap-py and you know it, clap your hands, (clap, clap) If you're

hap-py and you know it, then you real-ly ought to show it, If you're

hap-py and you know it clap your hands. (clap, clap)

Common Object Identification

Purpose:
- To develop awareness of the environment and the objects used in daily routines
- To develop communication skills
- To encourage appropriate social interaction
- To increase receptive language skills related to following simple directions

Materials:
- Bag of objects used in daily routines, such as brush, powder, soap, toothpaste, fork, napkin, comb, razor, tissue, shoestring, cup, pencil, keys, etc.

Preferred Setting:
Tabletop, or in the environments where the items are used.

Procedure:
1. Present an empty bag to the client.
2. Show and describe each item to the client as you place it in the bag. Talk about how, when, and where each item is used. When appropriate, demonstrate how to use the object.
3. Hand the bag to the client and encourage him/her to select an item. Provide physical assistance only when needed.
4. Question the individual about the item they selected, even if their developmental level suggests that they will have difficulty understanding the question or answering it. Continue to talk about the object. Ask the client to demonstrate the use of the object. Provide hand-over-hand assistance as needed.
5. Allow the individual ample opportunity to manipulate the object in his/her hands. Provide assistance as needed to insure a secure grasp of the object.
6. Encourage individuals to pass objects to other group members and to look at other group members who are using other items.
7. Continue this activity with other objects from the bag by using the same procedure.

Reminders:
Always encourage as much independence as possible. Assume that the individual may be able to understand what you are requesting or describing. If you expect more from people, often you receive a better response from them, and you discover abilities you never knew they had.

Find the Object

Purpose:
- To increase environmental awareness
- To increase knowledge of cause and effect
- To inspire curiosity

Materials:
- Windup objects (these are available commercially—see Part 3 for resources)
- One large scarf

Preferred Setting:
This scenario should be performed one to one on a tabletop. Both the client and caregiver need to be able to focus on the action with a minimum of distraction.

Procedure:
1. Place the windup object within the client's visual field, but outside their grasp.
2. Activate the object, paying close attention to see if the moving object appears to interest the client. Look for eye movements, attempts to reach out and catch the object, vocalizations, or any other movements/sounds that tell you there is some notice of the object. Reinforce any interaction with the object using both verbal and tactile praise.
3. Rewind the object.
4. As an alternative, before you activate the object, hold it in one hand and cover it with the scarf. Place the covered object in the person's visual field and let it go. If it falls off the table, let it go. (Sometimes clients have a stronger reaction to this than anything else.)

Reminders:
It is not difficult to find age-appropriate windup objects. There are objects in stores that are intended for adult collectors, including battery-operated objects.

Making Choices

Purpose:
- To enhance cognitive abilities (e.g., objective discrimination and identification)
- To increase exposure to cause/effect relationships, thus enhancing socialization skills
- To provide exposure to visual/tactile stimulation and discrimination through object exploration
- To enhance gross/fine motor skills (e.g., reaching, grasping) through tactile stimulation and manipulation of objects

Materials:
- Two to three food items (snacks, liquids, etc.)
- Two to three social/leisure objects (e.g., games, musical instruments, etc.)
- Two to three sensory objects (noisemakers, scented candles, neon-colored objects, etc.)
- Two to three items of clothing

Preferred Setting:
Tabletop. This activity will work best on an individual basis in an environment with minimal distractions.

Procedure:
1. Face the client, gaining his/her attention. This may be difficult, but it is necessary to begin this task.
2. In each open hand, show the client two items to be chosen. It is preferable to use two items of the same kind (two food items, two games, etc.).
3. Wait silently for the client to select one item. Many clients may attempt to collect both items; you should encourage the choice of only one item.
4. After a choice has been made, praise the client and use the word "Choice." ("Good choice!" "You chose the potato chips!," etc.)
5. Repeat this procedure using different sets of foods or other items.
6. For further practice, after a pattern has been set begin pairing a food item with a game. Continue to encourage the client to choose only one item.

Reminders:
1. When you first begin to use this scenario, use items for which the client(s) show a clear preference.
2. After preferences have been established, pair a highly preferred item with a less preferred item. (Not necessarily something the client hates but something that you know may not interest the client to a large degree.)
3. Eye contact is very important to the success of this scenario and should be maintained with the client as much as possible.

Memory Book

Purpose:
- To improve eye-hand coordination
- To assist in building meaningful relationships between events/ people/activities and their visual representations (e.g., photos, ribbons, greeting cards, etc.)
- To improve fine motor skills
- To provide visual stimulation
- To develop memory skills

Materials:
- Large scrapbook (these can be purchased or can be made from large pieces of construction paper or posterboard
- Glue sticks, tape, or any other adhesives
- Small personal mementos belonging to each client

Preferred Setting:
Tabletop

Procedure:
1. Gather all the materials and place them in front of each person in the group. Prior to working on each scrapbook, you should have a "show and tell" experience where each person's items are described to the other group members.
2. Explain the purpose of the activity to the group members.
3. Encourage each client to open their own scrapbook to the first clean page and to choose the first item to place in the book.
4. Encourage the client to apply tape or glue to that item, providing physical assistance only if necessary. If the client is only able to pick up the tape or glue and hand it to you, then encourage them to do that part of the task.
5. After the glue/tape is applied, assist the client in placing the memento in the book. Again, talk about the particular item and its connection to the person's life.
6. Repeat this process for each of the items. If you are working in a group, show and describe each item to all the group members so they are included while they are waiting for their turn. You could also consider having all the group members assist with the creation of one scrapbook.
7. Periodically, perhaps each week, add new items to the memory book as they become available. Take time to talk about both the new and older items and to look at previous pages in the book.

Reminders:
1. If you are having difficulty locating personal mementos, begin with pictures of favorite items or favorite people.
2. If you use background music to enhance this activity, choose instrumental music so the words of the songs do not compete with your talking.

Puzzles

Purpose:
- To encourage development of basic problem-solving skills
- To reinforce basic sequencing skills
- To increase eye-hand coordination
- To improve functional movements of hands/fingers
- To provide visual and tactile stimulation
- To provide an age-appropriate leisure experience

Materials:
- Age-appropriate puzzles that challenge cognitive and/or physical limitations (see Part 3 for ideas and resources)

Preferred Setting:
Tabletop

Procedure:
It is essential to consult the resource chapter of this book for ideas regarding the purchase or creation of AGE-APPROPRIATE puzzles. It is entirely possible to utilize the suggested resources to challenge the clients' developmental needs while ensuring the age-appropriateness of the activity:

1. Select a puzzle that fits the client's developmental level and also targets the preferences and interests of the person. If you are unable to determine preferences when you first begin the activity, you may notice a preference for a certain puzzle after several weeks or months. You may also have to modify a puzzle or use specialized adaptive puzzles based on physical or sensory challenges (see Part 3 for ideas).
2. It may be helpful to demonstrate how to complete/solve the puzzle. Demonstration often facilitates the performance of the individual.
3. Physical assistance may be needed for some individuals for successful manipulation of the puzzle pieces.
4. When you are completing the puzzle with the client, reinforce directional cues (e.g., "Take the piece out now"; "This piece goes underneath the other.")
5. Increasing the sensory feedback, especially visual, may promote greater independence. For example, you can outline both the puzzle piece, and the spot where it fits in the same color.
6. Encourage the clients' awareness of the puzzle's picture by describing it (talk about the actual picture, colors, shapes, etc.). You can include all group members in a discussion of one picture.

Reminders:
Always encourage as much independence as possible. Puzzle pieces can be as large as needed to promote client success.

CHAPTER 10

Communication

1. Story/Current Event Retelling

2. Taking Turns (Throwing a Ball)

3. Table Top Turn-Taking

4. Making Requests (Utilizing a Switch)

5. Adapted Yes/No Response

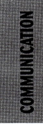

Story/Current Event Retelling

Purpose:
- To increase attending skills
- To acquaint clients with a controlled pre-literacy skill
- To increase exposure to auditory and visual stimuli
- To encourage socialization
- To promote fine motor skills (e.g., pointing, page turning)

Materials:
- Large books or magazines with pictures

Preferred Setting:
Tabletop, or other environment where reading or socialization naturally occurs (e.g., sitting on a sofa, or lying in bed). If you wish to promote optimal eye-hand use during this activity, it is recommended that the individual be seated in an upright position.

Procedure:
1. Explain to the clients that you are reading a story (talking about an event, etc.)
2. Provide the opportunity for each client to view the page and continue to do this throughout the activity.
3. Read the citation aloud one time.
4. Repeat the citation/text while pointing to the specific pictures as they are read.
5. Repeat the procedure for each page.
6. For each page, the reader may prompt each client to turn a page or the reader may prompt one client to turn all of the pages.
7. For each page, the reader may provide the least invasive prompt required to achieve a positive response for a client to identify a specific picture.

Reminders:
1. Try to maintain eye contact periodically with each client. This helps to increase their attention to the task.
2. Read at a slow pace. This will help you to relax and allows the opportunity for listeners to gain as much from the spoken language as possible.
3. Be as interactive as possible. Point to pictured objects in the book as you are reading. This will help to facilitate naming and identification.
4. Read something that is interesting to you. This will make the scenario less of a task. By using books that are interesting to you, the caregiver, the feedback you give to the client will be more interesting.

Taking Turns (Throwing a Ball)

Purpose:
- To learn to interact appropriately in a group using skills for taking turns
- To improve visual recognition skills
- To improve receptive language skills
- To learn to understand cause and effect through operation of a bladder device

Materials:
- Photographs of persons in the group
- 1-2-3 Baseball (See Part 3 for resources and explanation)
- A sign that says "Winner"

Preferred Setting:
If it is indoors, a large room is needed. If it is outdoors, an area with cement or a hard surface is needed.

Procedure:
1. Arrange clients in a circle.
2. Place the *1-2-3 Baseball* equipment on the floor and set it so that the ball can be thrown.
3. Place the bladder under the client's feet, in his/her hand, or on the wheelchair tray. Explain to the group that they are going to throw the ball by pushing on the bladder with their hands or feet. The person who throws the ball the farthest is the winner.
4. Shuffle through the photographs and hold one picture up. Name that person to the group and state that this is the person who will start the game.
5. Ask the first client to push the bladder switch to throw the ball, using only as much assistance as is necessary.
6. Measure the distance of the throw, then reset the ball.
7. Ask the first client to choose another person from the remaining photographs and to hold the picture up for everyone to see.
8. Repeat steps five, six, and seven until everyone has had a turn.
9. When the winner is determined, give the "Winner" card to that person and have him/her hold it up for everyone to see.

Reminders:
1. If the client is able to speak, he/should should be encouraged to say "My turn" and "Your turn" at the appropriate times. That person can also point to himself/herself and to a picture of the person whose turn is next.
2. The object of the game can be changed (e.g., throwing the ball into a basket).
3. If the client is unable to use hands or feet to operate the bladder, encourage him/her to use any body part they can, so they are as independent as possible.

Table Top Turn-Taking

Purpose:
- To teach a prerequisite communicative behavior
- To facilitate cause and effect behaviors through frequent practice and positive reinforcement
- To increase eye-hand coordination
- To facilitate socialization skills and abilities

Materials:
- One small to medium size ball, such as a nerf ball or kick ball. A medium-sized balloon may be substituted (See Part 3 for resources).

Preferred Setting:
Depending upon the type of table available, this scenario may be used with individuals or with groups of three (with a square-shaped table) or more (using an oval or half-moon shaped table). Two caregivers are required. The first caregiver is seated at the table, to roll the ball to each of the clients. The second caregiver is standing close to the clients to provide physical assistance (if necessary) for the clients to roll the ball back to the first caregiver.

Procedure:
For this scenario, the caregiver should sit at the head of the table with each of the clients involved seated at different edges of the table.

1. The lead caregiver is to call one of the clients to attention by calling his/her name.
2. If assistance is required to achieve this, the second caregiver should help focus the client's attention to the first caregiver, then to the ball.
3. The first caregiver then rolls the ball to the chosen client in a slow but steady motion.
4. The second caregiver then provides the lowest level of assistance required to help the client catch or otherwise get the ball, while he/she provides verbal praise upon receipt.
5. The first caregiver then verbally requests that the client roll the ball back to him/her.
6. The second caregiver then assists the client (using the least amount of assistance required) in rolling the ball back to the first caregiver, utilizing verbal praise throughout.
7. Repeat steps one through six with each person at the table.

Reminders:
1. Encourage independence as much as possible.
2. If you choose to use background music to facilitate movement and participation, use instrumental music. It can be confusing to clients to try to attend to your voice as well as to singing voices.

Making Requests (Utilizing a Switch)

Purpose:
- To reinforce goal attainment and communicative initiation skills
- To provide opportunities for real experiences in cause and effect

Materials:
- One BIGmack™ switch (See Part 3 for resource)
- Any objects or food items which the client finds desirable

Preferred Setting:
This scenario may be utilized in a variety of settings and can be adapted readily for small groups. It is ideal for one-on-one training as well as for group instruction.

Procedure:
1. Following the directions for the BIGmack™ switch, record a request message for the item chosen. For example: if the client likes cheese puffs, record a message like…"May I have some cheese puffs, please."
2. Sit across from the individual (tabletop or on the floor) and place both the switch and the desired item in a row. The switch must be positioned in front of the client, between the client and the desired item.
3. Prompt the client to activate the switch (following a prompting hierarchy from verbal to physical assistance). When you are prompting people, it is best to start with the least amount of prompting possible to see how much of the task they can do independently. Therefore, you should provide prompts in this order:
   a. Verbal (and if that does not work…)
   b. Gestural (pointing to the item)
   c. Tactile (touching the client, touching the item)
   d. Physical (hand over hand)

   After the switch has been activated the message will play.
4. Give the client a sample of the desired item and reinforce the exchange verbally, e.g., "Here you are; you really like these", etc.
5. Repeat steps one through four.

Reminders:
If the client can operate a tape recorder, this may be utilized instead of the BIGmack™ switch. The caregiver may find short playing message tapes at electronic stores.

Adapted Yes/No Response

Purpose:
- To facilitate cause and effect behaviors through frequent practice and positive reinforcement
- To improve both sound/symbol and sound/word relationships

Materials:
- Voice-output AAC (Augmentative/Alternative Communication) device is best. (The AAC device becomes a voice for the client.) These may be purchased relatively inexpensively from catalogs (see Part 3 for resources). For the device, two activation cells (buttons for different messages) are required.
- Samples of items that the client both likes and dislikes

Preferred Setting:
For this scenario, a one-to-one caregiver-client ratio is preferred. An environment free from unnecessary distractions is also preferable. This scenario may be completed both on a tabletop or on a rug.

Procedure:
1. Follow the directions for the chosen device and record "yes" for one cell and "no" for the other cell.
2. After the recording is completed, place "yes" and "no" signs on the corresponding cells.
3. Place the device between the client and you with "yes" and "no" facing the client.
4. Encourage the client to activate each cell, using the least amount of assistance necessary.
5. Place a desired item between the client and you (within the client's visual field).
6. Prompt the client to look at the desired item; ask the client "Would you like (desired item)?".
7. The client should have the opportunity to respond "yes"; you should wait for a response. If this does not occur independently, prompt the client to activate the "yes" cell with the least amount of assistance possible.
8. After the cell is activated, give the client the desired item and reinforce with verbal praise.
9. Repeat steps five through eight.
10. Repeat the same procedure for the "no" response. You will be using a nonpreferred item and removing it from the client after the "no" cell is activated.

Reminders:
1. Do not use items that are extremely negative to the client (for the "no" response). Try to use very desirable items for the "yes" response and more neutral items for the "no" response.

CHAPTER 11

Social/Recreation

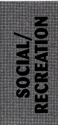

SOCIAL/RECREATION

Balloons and Music

Purpose:
• Increase socialization skills
• Increase peer awareness and relationships
• Increase eye-hand coordination
• Increase gross motor skills

Materials:
• Tape/CD Player and Preferred Music (Sedative is recommended.)
• Balloons (large and round)

Preferred Setting:
Seat the clients in two lines facing each other, an arm's length apart and about three feet across from each other (enough room for caregivers to stand next to clients to assist as needed).

Procedure:
1. Turn on tape/CD player (have one client operate this with a switch if you have one or assist the client in pushing the buttons).
2. Begin by standing in front of each client and tossing the balloon back and forth, encouraging the client either to hit it or catch it.
3. Encourage clients to toss the balloon back and forth to each other (it may take two caregivers to do this activity, one assisting each client in a pair). If necessary, use physical assistance.

Reminders:
1. Keep using the clients' names so the individuals become more aware of each other. Encourage clients to look at each other.
2. If you want to preserve balloons, keep them in a cool area. Heat will deflate them more quickly.
3. Do not do this activity with a large ball— they move too quickly.
4. Remember that the type of music used affects the mood of the activity. Sedative music is recommended because balloons move slowly and gently. However, you can use stimulative music if you are interested in a livelier activity.

Parachute

Purpose:
- To increase functional movements of arms
- To stimulate visually
- To increase socialization with caregivers and peers
- To increase responsiveness to the environment
- To maintain grasp of an object
- To increase participation in a group activity

Materials:
- Parachute (a sheet can also be used). Parachutes come in several sizes and can be purchased from catalogs (see Part 3 for resources)
- Foam ball(s) or balloon(s) placed in the center of the parachute
- Tape/CD player (optional)

Preferred Setting:
Clients should be seated in a circle in a large space. If possible, caregivers should be seated in this circle next to clients.

Procedure:
1. Clients should be seated in a circle that is the same size as the parachute.
2. Encourage clients to grasp the handles of the parachute or the edge of the parachute. Independence should be encouraged, and physical assistance should be used only if necessary.
3. Encourage clients to move the parachute in a variety of different ways: up and down, fast and slow, high and low, etc. Place the foam ball or balloon in the center and encourage clients to bounce it up and down.
4. Give the clients the opportunity to move their arms independently. Offer physical assistance only when difficulty arises.
5. Be creative with this activity and create your own movements. For example, you could have half of the circle moving the parachute up, while the other half moves it down, or you could put someone underneath the parachute in the middle of the circle and have the group lift the parachute over his/her head.

Reminders:
1. Begin the activity with only one ball or balloon in the center of the parachute. Add additional balls or balloons to increase the difficulty of the activity. Balloons should be used with clients who have slow movements or contractures because they move more slowly.
2. If you are using music, remember that the type of music you choose will affect the mood of the activity. If you want to talk during the activity, choose music that is instrumental only. If possible, have one client turn on the music.
3. Encourage clients to look at each other as they move the parachute.

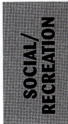

SOCIAL/
RECREATION

Shake Hands "Hello"

Purpose:
- Increase peer awareness and relationships
- Increase socialization skills
- Increase eye-hand coordination

Materials:
- None needed

Preferred Setting:
Any setting which allows the caregiver to greet the client face-to-face

Procedure:
The greeting song can be used to start any group or individual activity. It is an excellent way to provide a structured beginning and is useful because clients may learn to recognize this as such.

The greeting song can be any song the caregiver invents. Altering the words to songs that are well-known is often a good idea. Here is a suggestion:

To the tune of "Goodnight Ladies":
Hello Susan
Hello Susan
Hello Susan
How are you today? (or)
It's time say hello.
(This last line can be anything you need.)

After the song is completed, or during the singing of it, shake hands with the individual by first encouraging that person to reach out independently.

Reminders:
1. Make sure songs chosen are age-appropriate (i.e., do not use children's songs for adults).
2. Do not be shy about singing. Clients really enjoy it, and they certainly do not judge your abilities.
3. This same song can be used for a "Good bye," to close an activity.

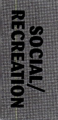

SOCIAL/ RECREATION

Play the Drum

Purpose:
- To develop awareness of peers
- To develop skills for taking turns
- To increase attention span
- To provide opportunities for gross motor movement

Materials:
- One drum and a mallet. There are many different varieties of drums. Ensure that the one you choose is appropriate for your clients. If they are capable of holding it up, you can choose a flatter style frame drum. If it is to be placed on a wheelchair tray, table, or floor, make sure it has a taller frame, so it will resonate when it is struck with the mallet. (See Part 3 for resources.) If necessary, the mallet handle can be adapted, so that clients can grasp it (See Part 3 for resources).

Preferred Setting:
Clients should be seated in a circle, so they can see one another. There should be enough room between clients (arm's length) so that caregivers have room to approach each person from the side.

Procedure:
1. Determine who will be the first person to play the drum; and, if possible, encourage that person to reach out to grasp both the drum and the mallet.
2. Encourage the client to play the drum as many times as he/she would like to (more than once or twice, if possible). Physically assist only if absolutely necessary. If the client is unable to use the mallet or appears to reject it, he/she can also play the drum with their bare hand.
3. Verbally direct all group members to listen and to look at whoever is playing the drum.
4. After the drum play is finished, encourage the client to pass the drum and mallet to the next person. Repeat these steps for each person.

Reminders:
Be aware that the use of background music could influence the way each client plays the drum. Decide whether you want to encourage a steady beat (to the background music) or free expression (no background music). Even at the profound level of mental retardation, some people may be able to keep a steady beat.

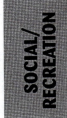

SOCIAL/ RECREATION

Tape/CD Player and Switch

Purpose:
- Attain a leisure skill
- Reinforce the concept of cause and effect
- Increase involvement and participation in a music activity

Materials:
- Tape/CD player
- Switch and Power Link® (see Part 3 for resources)
- Variety of tapes and/or CDs

Preferred Setting:
Tabletop or near a stereo system. This activity can be done with one individual in a small room or with one individual in a large group.

Procedure:
1. Determine the musical preference of the client (if possible) prior to teaching switch use.
2. Determine the best type of switch for each individual—there are many varieties that can be used, depending on each client's physical ability.
3. Demonstrate the use of the switch (i.e., each time the switch is used, the music comes on).
4. If necessary, physically assist the client in using the switch.
5. If you choose to reinforce this skill several times, the Power Link® can be set to stop the tape after a short period of time, such as three (3) minutes. The client then has to use the switch to keep re-activating the tape/CD player. The Power Link comes with easy instructions.)

Reminders:
1. If you plan to have music playing in your room, this is an excellent opportunity to have one individual turn it on.
2. The type of music played will affect the behavior of the clients (remember: stimulative vs sedative music discussed earlier). If this activity is being done with one client only, music should be the client's favorite.
3. If you use tapes, make sure they are cued to play exactly when the switch is activated. The client needs to understand immediate cause and effect.

Active Television Watching

Purpose:
- To increase basic social interaction skills and abilities
- To assist individuals with focusing and shifting attention
- To increase receptive vocabulary through a leisure activity
- To provide an age-appropriate leisure opportunity

Materials:
- TV and VCR
- Variety of videotapes. Choose tapes according to the preferences of the clients, but the following are also considered appropriate for this population: nature programs, musicals, music videos (especially country, gospel and rock), sports (especially ice skating, rhythmic gymnastics, surfing, skiiing, diving, track and field), dance videos (jazz, ballet), parade, and game shows (clients often attend to the electronic sounds, beeps, colors, etc.)

Preferred Setting:
This activity should occur in a room with few distractions. It should also have a television screen large enough for a group of people to watch simultaneously.

Procedure:
1. Encourage the client(s) to choose a tape and, if it is physically possible, to place it in the VCR.
2. If your television has an adaptive switch, encourage clients to turn on the television.
3. Prior to viewing, decide what you plan to focus on when you talk about the video (e.g., people, actions, colors, plot, etc.)
4. Using a moderate level of speech, alert clients to what they will be viewing.
5. Encourage a client to press "Play" on the remote.
6. As the tape progresses, point out anything that relates to the topic of focus. Periodically allow time for the clients to view the tape quietly, but spend more of your time directing their attention to what they are watching.

Reminders:
1. The goal of this activity is interaction, not looking at a videotape. Most tapes will probably surpass the clients' ability to comprehend, but these tapes will serve as a vehicle for attending, focusing, and interacting.
2. Be animated. Watching television is an interactive process. We all do things such as shouting during sports events or laughing during comedies. Demonstrate these emotions/actions for the clients. The more animated you are, the more interesting the activity will be.

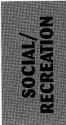

Board Games

Purpose:
- To provide age-appropriate leisure experiences
- To encourage socialization
- To improve functional movements of hands/fingers
- To improve eye-hand coordination
- To encourage completion of simple directions

Materials:
- There are age-appropriate board games that have been specifically manufactured for this population (See Part 3 for resources). Traditional board games can also be modified from their original form to meet cognitive or physical limitations.

Preferred Setting:
Tabletop

Procedure:
1. Seat the clients around the table facing each other and encourage their participation in the setup of the game using the least assistance possible (e.g., "Diane, can you take a card from the pack?" or "Judy, please pass a bingo card to Diane.").
2. Each client should have the opportunity physically to participate during their turn at their level of competence, if possible. Verbal directions should reflect the possible need to break each step into its smallest components to ensure client success. For example, you might need to say "Mark, it is your turn to pick up a checker. Mark, pick up the red checker. Mark, place the red checker on the red square." It is possible that Mark might be able to pick up the checker independently, but he might need physical assistance with the rest of his turn.
3. Ensure that each client has the opportunity to take several turns until the game is completed. For each step, try to increase the level of participation and include such actions as:
   a. "Look at the _____."
   b. "Pick up the _____."
   c. "Place the _____."
   d. "Pass the _____ to Mark."
   Always encourage clients to watch others as they take turns in the game.
4. When the game is completed, involve the clients in the task of putting away materials.

Reminders:
1. If clients are visually impaired, increase the use of verbal cues and tactile assistance. Ensure that people with visual difficulties have the opportunity for orientation to the sizes, shapes and location of game pieces.

Plant Care

Purpose:
- To provide opportunities for an age-appropriate leisure activity
- To provide an opportunity to assume a caregiver role
- To improve the functional movements of arms
- To improve bilateral use of arms
- To improve eye-hand coordination
- To gain exposure to a variety of visual and tactile sensory stimuli
- To encourage the following of verbal directions

Materials:
- Seeds, seedlings, or mature plants
- Supplies related to specific plant care activities (handheld shovel for transplanting, scissors for trimming, watering can, hose, etc.)

Preferred Setting:
This activity should take place in the environment where plant care would occur naturally (e.g., windowsill area, tabletop). Plant care should also take place outside, if possible. You might consider creating an elevated garden that could easily be reached by people using wheelchairs.

Procedure:
1. Place all the materials on the table and describe each item to the members of the group.
2. If you are beginning with planting seeds (as opposed to caring for a mature plant), encourage each client to choose seeds to plant. If you have seed packets with colorful pictures, this may elicit a choice.
3. If you are beginning with transplanting seedlings, it will be more difficult to make choices, because all the plants will look similar at this stage. You could still encourage choices from the pictures on the pack-

ets, and then place that particular plant in front of the client.
4. Demonstrate each step of the planting procedure as you encourage clients to participate. Use physical assistance only if necessary. If you find that clients are skilled at one particular aspect of the task, you might want to work in assembly line fashion, as you continue to plant more seeds during this activity or on other days. The planting activity can be subdivided as follows:
   a. Open the seed packet.
   b. Pour seeds from the packet into a person's hand or a dish.
   c. Transfer potting soil from the bag into the pot.
   d. Poke a hole in the center of the dirt using a pencil or similar item.
   e. Place several seeds in the hole and cover with dirt.
   f. Fill the watering can with water.
   g. Water the seeds.
5. During the planting process, describe the various tasks in terms of textures, scents, etc. Ensure that clients have ample opportunity for maximum sensory input.
6. After the planting is completed, assist the clients with placing their plants in the appropriate spot for the type of light they need. Explain this procedure to the clients.
7. Set up a watering schedule for the clients to follow. Organize a plant growth chart as well. The clients should interact with their plants every day, providing water and/or checking for growth. When it is time to transplant, follow the same procedure stated above.

Reminders:
1. Plants need to be cared for on a daily basis, and it is important to include the clients in this daily care.
2. This activity can be done outside as well as inside. You can include other plant care activities in your daily routine, such as watering flowers with a sprayer hose, pruning bushes, and trimming vines.

Pet Care

Purpose:
- To provide an age-appropriate leisure opportunity
- To encourage physical expressions of affection
- To provide an opportunity to assume a caregiver role
- To practice related self-help skills (e.g., feeding, bathing, grooming)
- To improve functional movement of arms

Materials:
- Supplies related to specific pet care activity (e.g., comb/brush, ball or play toy, soap, towels, grooming mitt). If needed, the handle of the comb or brush can be adapted for client use (see Part 3 for suggestions)
- Pet treats (edibles)

Preferred Setting:
The authors emphasize utilizing this scenario in the environment where this particular activity occurs normally (e.g., bathroom for bathing, and kitchen for feeding). If this is a group activity, find a larger area still naturally suitable for the activity.

Procedure:
For the purposes of this procedure we will address "grooming a dog", but these steps and ideas can be applied to any aspect of pet care.

1. Place the grooming materials in front of the client so he or she can select a brush. Physically assist the client only if necessary. If you need an adaptive handle, ensure that this is available.
2. Demonstrate how to brush the animal's coat.
3. Encourage the client to brush the animal the same way you just did. Physically assist as needed, but allow the client as much independence as possible. It may be necessary to allow some time for the client to simply touch the pet first and/or to watch its behavior.
4. As you groom the dog, talk to the client about what you are doing and why. Talk about the characteristics of the animal.
5. When grooming is completed, encourage the client to give the dog a treat and to praise the dog (verbally or by petting).

Reminders:
1. Ensure that the pet is situated within the range of motion of the client. Consult with an occupational therapist or physical therapist if you are uncertain about the physical capabilities of the clients.
2. Ensure that the animal chosen is not aggressive in any way, enjoys being groomed, and will not cause any allergic reactions.
3. If a dog is unavailable at your home or facility, consider contacting the local humane society or a pet therapy organizaion.

Part Three

Materials and Resources

Scenario Specific Materials Including Catalogs and Books

This chapter provides resources for the materials recommended in each scenario. This may consist of information on purchasing and/or instructions on "making your own." For some activities the use of a particular product will be recommended; in most cases effective alternatives have been found. For those scenarios that utilize common household or workroom items, there will be no recommendations. For easy references, scenarios are listed in the order in which they appear in this book.

ACTIVITIES OF DAILY LIVING

MUSIC ASSISTED PERSONAL GROOMING
No recommendations.

SKIN CARE
No recommendations.

HAIR CARE
Search "Activities of Daily Living Products" on the internet

PREDRESSING SKILLS
No recommendations.

ADAPTIVE FASTENER FRAMES
Catalog: Sammons Preston
www.sammonspreston.com

Create your own: you will need wood, fabric, nails or wood glue, and the desired fasteners.

MEAL PREPARATION
Catalog: Flaghouse: Special Populations
601 Flaghouse Drive
Haskbrouck Heights, NJ 07604
800-793-7900
www.flaghouse.com

S & S adaptAbility
75 Mill Street
P.O. Box 513
Colchester, CT 06415-0513
800-226-8856
www.ssww.com

BEVERAGE PREPARATION
Catalogs: S & S adaptAbility
75 Mill Street
P.O. Box 513
Colchester, CT 06415-0513
800-226-8856

Search "Activities of Daily Living" on the internet

HOMEMAKING
Catalog: Sammons Preston
www.sammonspreston.com

ACTIVITIES OF DAILY LIVING (continued)

USING SWITCHES
Catalogs: AbleNet, Inc.
2808 Fairview Ave.
Roseville, MN, 55113-1308
800-322-0956
(for PowerLink® and BIGmack™)
www.ablenetinc.com

Enabling Devices
Toys for Special Children
385 Warburton Avenue
Hasting-on-Hudson, NY 10706
800-832-8697
www.enablingdevices.com

Create your own:
Book: *Homemade Battery-Powered
Toys and Educational Devices for
Severely Handicapped Children*
by Linda Burkhart
(available from author)
8503 Rhode Island Avenue
College Park, MD 20740

SENSORY STIMULATION

AROMAS
Catalog: Flaghouse: Special Populations
601 Flaghouse Drive
Haskbrouck Heights, NJ 07604
800-793-7900
www.flaghouse.com

NATURE BOX
No recommendations.

DARK BOX/COLUMN
Create your own: You will need a portable
space. You can use a very large box, such as
a shipping box from a large appliance. Paint
the inside black, or line with black material
or paper. The box must be completely dark,
with no light inside.

FIND THE MUSICAL SOUND
Catalogs: Music Is Elementary
P.O. Box 24263
Cleveland, OH 44124
800-888-7502
www. musiciselementary.com

West Music Company
P.O. Box 5521
1208 5th Street
Coralville, IA 52241
800-397-9378
www.westmusic.com

FIND THE SOUND
No recommendations.

SENSORY STIMULATION (continued)

**MUSIC—PLAYING RHYTHM
INSTRUMENTS**
Catalogs: Music Is Elementary
P.O. Box 24263
Cleveland, OH 44124
800-888-7502
www. musiciselementary.com

West Music Company
P.O. Box 5521
1208 5th Street
Coralville, IA 52241
800-397-9378

Create your own:
Book: *Clinically Adapted Instruments for
the Multiple Handicapped*
Compiled by Cynthia Clark and
Donna Chadwick

In addition, you can make your own
instruments. Some examples are:
Drum: Use pots and pans with spoons for
mallets.
Sandblocks: Use sandpaper pasted on blocks
of wood.
Shakers/Maracas: Put rice or dried beans,
etc., in empty cans and tape the opening.
You can also use pill bottles, small jars,
plastic eggs, small plastic soda bottles—
any small receptacle. If the shaker is clear,
you can add visual stimuli such as glitter,
scraps of colored paper and colored beads.
Banjo: Use a cigar box with rubber bands
stretched across it.
Tambourine: Drive a nail through two or
three bottle caps and nail this onto a small
piece of wood. The bottle caps need to
move freely against each other when the
wood is moved back and forth.

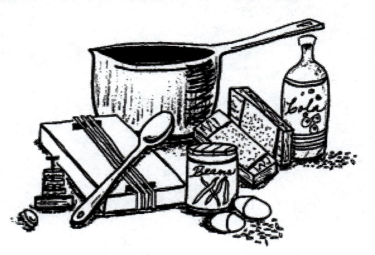

MUSIC AND TACTILE DEFENSIVENESS
No recommendations.

VIBRATION (SNAKES AND TUBES)
Catalog: Flaghouse: Special Populations
601 Flaghouse Drive
Haskbrouck Heights, NJ 07604
800-793-7900
www.flaghouse.com

TEXTURE RUB
No recommendations.

BRUSHING
No recommendations.

DEEP MASSAGE
No recommendations.

WATER EXPLORATION
No recommendations.

SPONGES
No recommendations.

WALKING
No recommendations.

GROSS MOTOR

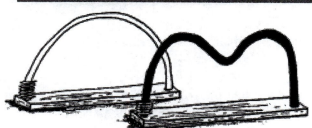

SHOULDER ARC
Catalogs: S & S adaptAbility
75 Mill Street
P.O. Box 513
Colchester, CT 06415-0513
800-226-8856
www.ssww.com

Create your own: You will need a wood base, and you will attach half of a hula hoop (or anything else that will create an arc. You could use PVC if you can find rings that will go around its diameter). For the rings—use children's plastic bracelets, plastic rings from children's toys, or cut holes in plastic lids.

MOVEMENT WITH RIBBON STICKS OR SCARVES
Catalogs: S & S adaptAbility
75 Mill Street
P.O. Box 513
Colchester, CT 06415-0513
800-226-8856
www.ssww.com

West Music Company
P.O. Box 5521
1208 5th Street
Coralville, IA 52241
800-397-9378
www.westmusic.com

Create your own: Ribbon sticks can be made by taking five or six very thin satin ribbons, multicolored, and attaching them to the tip of a wide dowel stick with a sturdy thumb tack. The stick can be painted bright colors.

"PLAY THE XYLOPHONE"
Catalogs: West Music Company
P.O. Box 5521
1208 5th Street
Coralville, IA 52241
800-397-9378
www.westmusic.com

Music Is Elementary
P.O. Box 24263
Cleveland, OH 44124
800-888-7502
www. musiciselementary.com

These instruments will be expensive, but are worth the price. Do not substitute children's xylophones—you will sacrifice quality and sound.

HOKEY POKEY
Recording: *The Hokey Pokey and Other Favorites*
Melody House Publishing Company
819 North West 92nd
Oklahoma City, OK 73114

Create your own: You could make a tape of anyone singing the Hokey Pokey. This is recommended, because you can choose your particular dance movements and also the speed of the song.

DANCE/MOVEMENT WITH CHINESE JUMPROPE
Catalog: Sportime Abilitations
800-850-8603
(Order a "Co-oper Band™")
www.abilitations.com

Create your own: Chinese jumpropes can be purchased in toy stores, or you can make a stretchy loop with wide elastic covered with a soft, pliable material.

GROSS MOTOR (continued)

THERAPY BALLS

Catalogs: Sportime Abilitations
800-850-8603
(Order a "Co-oper Band™")
www.abilitations.com

Flaghouse: Special Populations
601 Flaghouse Drive
Haskbrouck Heights, NJ 07604
800-793-7900
www.flaghouse.com

BEANBAG "BASKETBALL"

Catalogs: Music Is Elementary
P.O. Box 24263
Cleveland, OH 44124
800-888-7502
www. musiciselementary.com

West Music Company
P.O. Box 5521
1208 5th Street
Coralville, IA 52241
800-397-9378
www.westmusic.com

Create your own: Beanbags are easy to
make. Buy dried beans in the supermarket.
Sew the beans into small material sacks.
You should choose a heavy quality material.

OBSTACLE COURSE

No recommendations.

FINE MOTOR

THERAPEUTIC PUTTY

Catalog: Sammons Preston
www.sammonspreston.com

Create your own:
Basic recipe—
1 cup flour
1 cup salt
1/2 cup water
Dry tempera powder (any color)
Mix flour, salt and water in bowl. If too
gooey, add more flour. Sprinkle tempera on
dough (for color) and blend well. This will
air-dry in two to four days. Keeps up to
three weeks, refrigerated, in plastic bag.
Keeps one week unrefrigerated.

SANDBOX

No recommendations.

MANIPULATION BOX

Catalogs: Music Is Elementary
P.O. Box 24263
Cleveland, OH 44124
800-888-7502
www. musiciselementary.com

West Music Company
P.O. Box 5521
1208 5th Street
Coralville, IA 52241
800-397-9378
www.westmusic.com

FINE MOTOR (continued)

EGG SHAKER CHANT
Catalogs: Music Is Elementary
P.O. Box 24263
Cleveland, OH 44124
800-888-7502
www. musiciselementary.com

West Music Company
P.O. Box 5521
1208 5th Street
Coralville, IA 52241
800-397-9378
www.westmusic.com

Create your own: you can make egg shakers from the plastic eggs often sold at the Easter holiday. These can be filled with dried beans or rice or small hard items. These will not have the same weight and quality as those commercially available, which are inexpensive.

MAGNETS
No recommendations.

PEG BOARD
Catalog: Sammons Preston
www.sammonspreston.com

Create your own: Drill holes in a piece of wood and create pegs from dowels or other objects that will fit in the holes.

BRIGHT BUILDERS
Catalogs: S & S adaptAbility
75 Mill Street
P.O. Box 513
Colchester, CT 06415-0513
800-226-8856
www.ssww.com

CONTAINERS
No recommendations.

LOCK BOARD
Catalogs: S & S adaptAbility
75 Mill Street
P.O. Box 513
Colchester, CT 06415-0513
800-226-8856
www.ssww.com

COLLAGES
Catalog: Sammons Preston
www.sammonspreston.com
(for adapted sissors)

STAMP COLLECTION
No recommendations.

FLOWER ARRANGING
No recommendations.

PREWRITING
Catalog: www.doverpublications.com

COGNITIVE

ENVIRONMENTAL SOUNDS TAPE

Catalogs: Enabling Devices
           Toys for Special Children
           385 Warburton Avenue
           Hasting-on-Hudson, NY 10706
           800-832-8697
           enablingdevices.com

           AbleNet, Inc.
           2808 Fairview Ave.
           Roseville, MN, 55113-1308
           800-322-0956
           www.ablenetinc.com

IMITATION
No recommendations.

BODY PARTS IDENTIFICATION
No recommendations.

MUSIC AND MOVEMENT:
"IF YOU'RE HAPPY AND YOU KNOW IT"
No recommendations.

FIND THE OBJECT
No recommendations.

MAKING CHOICES
No recommendations.

PUZZLES

Catalogs: Flaghouse: Special Populations
           601 Flaghouse Drive
           Haskbrouck Heights, NJ 07604
           800-793-7900
           www.flaghouse.com

           Age Appropriate Resources
           T.F.H. (USA) Ltd.
           4537 Gibsonia Road
           Gibsonia, PA 15044
           800-467-6222
           www.tfhusa.com

Create your own: You can make puzzles by glueing a picture or photo on cardboard and cutting it into large shapes. This can also be done with the wood.

An easy alternative is purchasing plastic placemats and cutting them into large shapes. You could also put together a standard 500 or 1000 piece puzzle, break it up into large segments, and glue these segments on a backing.

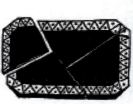 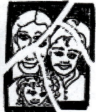

COMMUNICATION

STORY/CURRENT EVENT RETELLING
No recommendations.

TAKING TURNS (THROWING A BALL)
After extensive research, the only object which could be found to throw a ball at a reasonable rate is a children's toy called "1-2-3 Baseball". This is available at toy stores and is made by Playskool.

TAKING TURNS (TABLE TOP)
Catalog: Flaghouse: Special Populations
601 Flaghouse Drive
Haskbrouck Heights, NJ 07604
800-793-7900
www.flaghouse.com

MAKING REQUESTS (UTILIZING A SWITCH)
Catalogs: Enabling Devices
Toys for Special Children
385 Warburton Avenue
Hasting-on-Hudson, NY 10706
800-832-8697
enablingdevices.com

AbleNet, Inc.
2808 Fairview Ave.
Roseville, MN, 55113-1308
800-322-0956
www.ablenetinc.com

ADAPTED YES/NO RESPONSE
Catalogs: Enabling Devices
Toys for Special Children
385 Warburton Avenue
Hasting-on-Hudson, NY 10706
800-832-8697
enablingdevices.com

Mayer-Johnson Co.
P.O. BOx 1579
Solana Beach, CA 92075-1579
800-588-4548
www. mayer-johnson.com

SOCIAL/RECREATION

BALLOONS AND MUSIC
No recommendations.

PARACHUTE
Catalog: Flaghouse: Special Populations
601 Flaghouse Drive
Haskbrouck Heights, NJ 07604
800-793-7900
www.flaghouse.com

SHAKE HANDS "HELLO"
No recommendations.

PLAY THE DRUM
Catalogs: West Music Company
P.O. Box 5521
1208 5th Street
Coralville, IA 52241
800-397-9378
www.westmusic.com

Remo, Inc.
28101 Industry Dr.
Valencia, CA 91355
661-294-5600
www. remo.com

Create your own: If your clients need a built-up adapted handle for the mallet, an inexpensive method is to purchase pipe insulation 3/8" from a hardware store and cut it into smaller pieces. The hole will be too wide for the mallet handle, but you can wrap the handle with masking tape until it fits the pipe insulation. This is much less expensive than buying therapeutic built-up foam.

TAPE/CD PLAYER AND SWITCH
Catalog: AbleNet, Inc.
2808 Fairview Ave.
Roseville, MN, 55113-1308
800-322-0956
www.ablenetinc.com

ACTIVE TELEVISION WATCHING
No recommedations.

BOARD GAMES
Catalogs: Flaghouse: Special Populations
601 Flaghouse Drive
Haskbrouck Heights, NJ 07604
800-793-7900
www.flaghouse.com

Age Appropriate Resources
T.F.H. (USA) Ltd.
4537 Gibsonia Road
Gibsonia, PA 15044
800-467-6222
www.tfhusa.com

PLANT CARE
No recommendations.

PET CARE
Search "Activities of Daily Living" on the internet.

Bibliography & Recommended Reading

Alberto, P., Jobes, N., Sizemore, A., & Doran, D.A. (1980). A comparison of individual and group instruction across response tasks. *Journal of the Association for the Severely Handicapped,* 5, 285-293.

American Psychiatric Association. (1994). *Diagnostic and statistical manual of mental disorders.* (4th ed.). Washington, D.C.: Author.

Beukelman, D.R. & Mirenda, P. (1992). *Augumentative and alternative communication: management of severe communication disorders in children and adults.* Baltimore: Paul H. Brookes.

Bourland, G., Jablonski, E., & Lockhart, D. (1988). Multiple-behavior comparison of group and individual instruction of persons with mental retardation.l *Mental Retardation* 26(1), 39-46.

Boxill, E.H. (1985). *Music therapy for the developmentally disabled.* Rockville: Aspen Systems

Bruscia, K.E. (1989). *Defining music therapy.* Phoenixville, PA: Barcelona. 2nd edition—1998

Clair, A.A. (1996). *Therapeutic uses of music with older adults.* Baltimore: Health Professions

Favell, J.E., & McGimsey, J.F. (1978). Relative effectiveness and efficiency of group versus individual training of severely retarded persons. *American Journal of Mental Deficiency* 83, 104-109.

Fine, A., Welch-Burke, C., & Fondario, L. (1985). A developmental model for re-integration of leisure programming in the education of individuals with mental retardation. *Mental Retardation* 23(6), 289-296.

Gardner, J. & Chapman, M. (1990). *Program issues in developmental disabilities: a guide to effective habilitation and active treatment,* (2d ed). Baltimore: Paul H. Brookes

Garrett, B.A. & Greenwald, N.F. (1994). *Nonverbal interaction with adult clients: strategies for caregivers.* Tucson: Therapy Skill Builders.

Gaston, E.T. (1968). *Music in therapy.* New York: MacMillan.

Hanser, S.B. (1987). *Music therapist's handbook.* St. Louis: Warren H. Green. 2nd edition—1999

Horton, S. & Taylor, D. (1989). The use of behavior therapy and physical therapy to promote independent ambulation in a pre-schooler with mental retardation and cerebral palsy. *Research in Developmental Disabilities,* 10, 363-375.

Kielhofner, G. (Ed.), (1985). *A model of human occupation: theory and application.* Baltimore: Williams and Wilkins.

Manfredini, D. & Smith, W. (1988). The concept and implementation of active treatment. In *Community residences for persons with developmental disabilities: here to stay.* M. Janicki & M.W. Krauss (eds.), Baltimore: Paul H. Brookes.

Matson, T. Sadowski, C., Matese M., & Benavidez, D. (1993). Emipirical Study of mental health profession' knowledge and attitudes towards the concept of age-appropriateness. *Mental Retardation,* 31(5), 340-345.

Orelove, F.P. & Sobsey, D. (1987). *Educating children with multiple disabilities: A transdisciplinary approach.* Baltimore: Paul H. Brookes.

Rainforth, B., York, J., & McDonald, C. (1992). *Collaborative teams for students with severe disabilities: integrating therapy and educational services.* Baltimore: Paul H. Brookes.

Storm, R.H. & Willis, J.H. (1978). Small-group training as an alternative to individual programs for profoundly retarded persons. *American Journal of Mental Deficiency,* 83, 283-288.

Tannen, D. (1990). *You just don't understand women and men in conversation.* New York: Merrow.